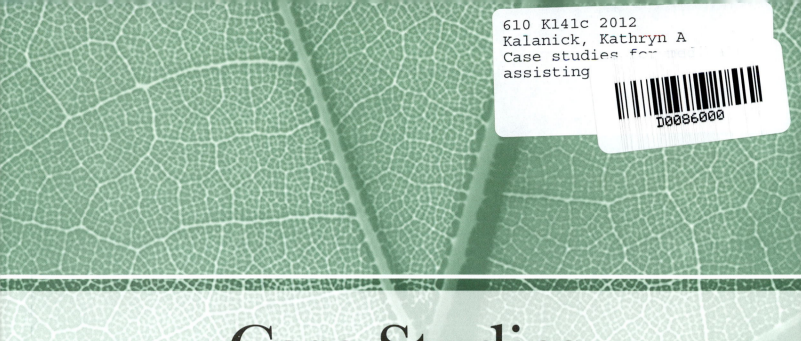

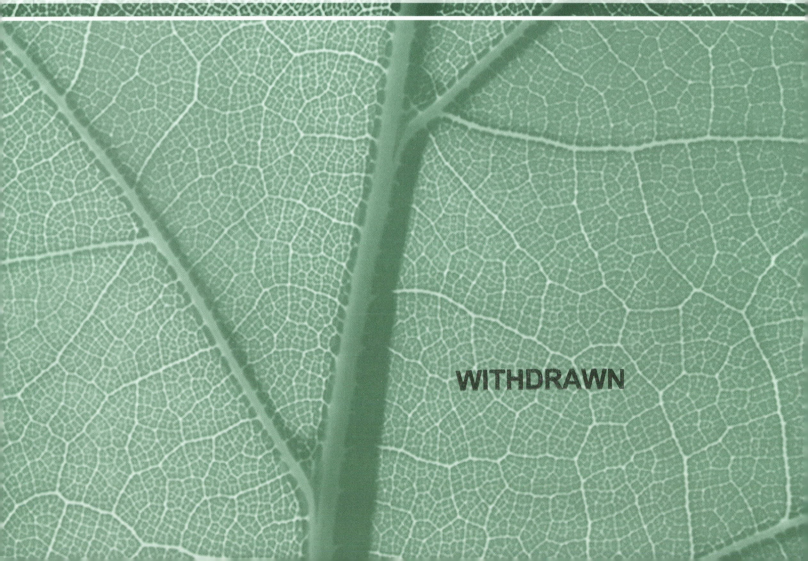

Case Studies
for Medical Assisting

Case Studies
for Medical Assisting

Kathryn A. Kalanick

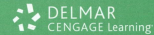

DELMAR
CENGAGE Learning·

Australia • Canada • Mexico • Singapore • Spain • United Kingdom • United States

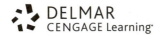

Case Studies for Medical Assisting,
Kathryn A. Kalanick

Vice President, Careers & Computing: Dave Garza

Director of Learning Solutions: Matthew Kane

Executive Editor: Rhonda Dearborn

Managing Editor: Marah Bellegarde

Senior Product Manager: Sarah Prime

Product Manager: Lauren Whalen

Vice President, Marketing: Jennifer Ann Baker

Marketing Director: Wendy E. Mapstone

Senior Marketing Manager: Nancy Bradshaw

Marketing Coordinator: Piper Huntington

Production Director: Wendy Troeger

Production Manager: Andrew Crouth

Design and Project Management:
S4Carlisle Publishing Services

For product information and technology assistance, contact us at
Cengage Learning Customer & Sales Support, 1-800-354-9706
For permission to use material from this text or product,
submit all requests online at **www.cengage.com/permissions.**
Further permissions questions can be e-mailed to
permissionrequest@cengage.com

Library of Congress Control Number: 2012941796

ISBN-13: 978-1-4354-3844-6

ISBN-10: 1-4354-3844-2

Delmar
5 Maxwell Drive
Clifton Park, NY 12065-2919
USA

Cengage Learning is a leading provider of customized learning solutions with office locations around the globe, including Singapore, the United Kingdom, Australia, Mexico, Brazil, and Japan. Locate your local office at:
international.cengage.com/region

Cengage Learning products are represented in Canada by Nelson Education, Ltd.

To learn more about Delmar, visit **www.cengage.com/delmar**

Purchase any of our products at your local college store or at our preferred online store **www.cengagebrain.com**

Notice to the Reader
Publisher does not warrant or guarantee any of the products described herein or perform any independent analysis in connection with any of the product information contained herein. Publisher does not assume, and expressly disclaims, any obligation to obtain and include information other than that provided to it by the manufacturer. The reader is expressly warned to consider and adopt all safety precautions that might be indicated by the activities described herein and to avoid all potential hazards. By following the instructions contained herein, the reader willingly assumes all risks in connection with such instructions. The publisher makes no representations or warranties of any kind, including but not limited to, the warranties of fitness for particular purpose or merchantability, nor are any such representations implied with respect to the material set forth herein, and the publisher takes no responsibility with respect to such material. The publisher shall not be liable for any special, consequential, or exemplary damages resulting, in whole or in part, from the readers' use of, or reliance upon, this material.

Printed in the United States of America
1 2 3 4 5 6 7 16 15 14 13 12

Dedication

This book is dedicated to every student who has touched my life and taught me the true meaning and value of education.

This book is also dedicated to my favorite student, and my favorite medical assistant, who just happens to be my beautiful daughter, Andrea King. Without your love and support, your suggestions for names and scenarios, and your availability for middle-of-the-night long-distance phone calls, I would still be toiling away on the first draft. Your knowledge, expertise, and generous spirit have been priceless.

Words of Gratitude

This book has been a labor of love for a profession that is near and dear to my heart. I will be forever grateful to my colleague, Bradley Moore, for encouraging me to think outside the proverbially box and for not taking "maybe" for an answer. I am equally grateful to a wonderful group of instructors and students at Remington College's Nashville campus who agreed to take two days out of their lives, five years ago, to allow me the privilege to test-drive this project.

I would like to express my gratitude to my editor, Rhonda Dearborn, senior product manager, Sarah Prime, and Bev Kraus, project manager at S4Carlisle Publishing Services—their encouragement, professionalism, and commitment have been invaluable. A special thank you goes out to the rest of the development team: your worth is immeasurable.

I feel so blessed to have such wonderful reviewers. Their insight, perspective, criticisms, suggestions, and tremendous knowledge have truly enhanced this textbook.

I would also like to thank four amazing medical professionals, Marc Jones, DO, and his medical assistant, Shawnna Carter, for answering my technical questions and verifying dosages, tests, procedures, and treatment plans and Kimberly Hockaday, NCMA, NCET, NCICS, Program Director, Medical Assisting & Medical Billing and Coding Carrington College and Erika Breitwieser Medical Assisting instructor for Carrington College for their input and advice in completing insurance resource documents.

And, most importantly, thank you to my husband, Geno, my children, grandchildren, and my mother. Without their support, encouragement, and patience this project would not have been possible.

Contents

Part 1   Case Studies 1

Clinical Case Studies

Comprehensive Case Studies

Part 2   Rubrics. 163

Preface

The concept of teaching through case studies is not new. From my very first class, 30 years ago, to my last class, I have used case studies in one form or another to augment my lesson plans. Case studies can be found in almost every textbook, regardless of the discipline. We have all spent time writing a case study or two, and we have conjured them out of thin air on the spot to illustrate a point or provide an example. But now more than ever, we *need* to teach through case studies. Long gone are the days we could stand in front of the class and lecture for hours. Gone, too, are the days we could simply assign our students a case study at the end of a chapter to read and answer a few questions.

Today's students need to be actively engaged 100% of the time. They need to live it—breathe it—and own it. As educators, we may struggle against this or we can embrace it.

Let's look at some of the dynamics of the contemporary student in Table FM-1.

TABLE FM-1   Dynamics of the Contemporary Student

Personality	• Has a drive to achieve
	• Is optimistic
	• Feels special; student has been treated as if he or she is special all of his or her life
	• Is highly protected (overindulgent parents)
	• Has an expectation that his or her parents, college advisors, or instructors will resolve his or her conflicts
	• Is motivated, goal oriented, assertive, and confident
	• Wants to make a difference
	• Is conventional
	• Is respectful to adults
	• Values manners
	• Is more accepting of lifestyle, racial, and ethnic differences
Information Processing	• Studies less (this applies to students of all ability levels; a decline in the past five years)
	• Feels pressured to succeed, high achieving
	• Has had more homework than previous generations
	• Is efficient at multitasking and believes it is the smart thing to do (although he or she has challenges with time management)
	• Has *zero* tolerance for delays and idle time
	• Does not want to sit and listen to lectures hours on end
Social Interaction	• Spends more time social networking
	• Is team oriented
	• Needs constant contact with peers

Thus, instructional methods that reach contemporary students:

- Provide clear expectations
- Provide detailed instructions
- Create explicit syllabi
- Use technology as much as possible (as long as it is applicable)
- Use social networking as often as possible
- Embrace alternate ways of doing things

According to Neil Howe, speaker and best-selling author of *Millennials Go to College: Strategies for a New Generation on Campus,* successful instructional methods include:

- Emphasize teamwork and assign group projects
- Service learning—community service
- Prepare for students who have a lot and expect a lot
- Stress good outcomes
- Use social norming
- Create expectations for success
- Stress friendship and duty to others
- Retool classrooms for constant feedback
- Monitor skill mastery
- Expect students to be more knowledgeable and less creative

Interactive Learning Environment

"An interactive classroom is one in which students participate as equal partners in an ongoing discovery process."

—Adam Allerhand, Professor at Indiana University

Let's talk about retooling the classroom for constant feedback, creating the interactive classroom that the contemporary student all but demands.

A colleague of mine asked me what I thought about teaching an entire clinical course by using case studies only. My first thought was that it couldn't be done (and I believe I said as much). He encouraged me to "just think about it for awhile." So I did, and I became so interested in the concept that I asked my medical assistant instructors at a staff meeting to pick one topic that they had not previously addressed and teach it only through case studies and role-play. I even went so far as to have them give their students the same written examination they would have given them had they only lectured the topic and report back the following week. The experiment was a huge success. ***Every instructor reported back that his or her students had*** *far exceeded the instructor's expectations and that not one student had failed the written examination* (the instructors had been prepared to lecture the material and allow the students to retest).

However, it took quite a bit of time for the instructors to create the case studies and orchestrate them in the classroom. They thought it was fun and educational, but none of them wanted to spend the time to expand on it further.

Contemporary Case Studies

My colleague and I later discussed the potential of teaching only through case studies in depth, the pros and cons, the level of detail that would be required. Was it even possible? This led to what I am calling the *contemporary case study*.

"The contemporary case study requires a more detailed scenario, active participation, and a component of research. It also requires a demonstration of competencies, professional documentation, and professional communication."

The contemporary case study can sustain 80% to 100% of a course grade and provide the basis for grade assignation. Grades must be assigned for completion of task and correct response. Soft skills are also subtly addressed throughout each case study. Group interaction and peer mentoring are essential. Table FM-2 compares traditional case studies with contemporary case studies.

TABLE FM-2   Traditional versus Contemporary Case Studies

Traditional Case Studies	Contemporary Case Studies
Brief scenario: two to four sentences	Detailed scenario: two or more paragraphs
Read and respond to one to four questions	Participation required; may include:
	One to six questions
	Brief research paper
	Professional documentation and communication
	Research and role-play scenario
	Ability to demonstrate competencies
Graded for completion–correct answer	Basis for grade assignation may include:
	Completion
	Correct response
	Ability to demonstrate competencies
	Appropriate interpersonal interactions
Nominal percentage of grade	Majority of grade percentage: 80–100%
Limited application of skills	Ability to demonstrate competencies

© Cengage Learning 2013

Benefits of Case Studies

The benefits of using a contemporary case study, either individually or as part of an overall teaching experience, are innumerable, and include:

- Enhanced learning environment
- Application of skills

- Hands-on experience
- Preparation for employment
- Complete enactment of competencies

Case Study Design

- **Two-hour block application.** Contemporary case studies work best when written for a two-hour block of time. Anything less would be insufficient to address a situation properly.

- **Multiple skills introduced in each case study.** Multiple skills should be incorporated; for example, when a medical assistant takes a patient back to an examination room, he or she isn't *just* taking that patient's vital signs. Professional communication skills, patient assessment skills, and appropriate documentation skills are also employed.

- **All competencies are covered.** CAHAAP, ABHES, and NCCT competencies are addressed in the case studies.

- **Use individually or together to strengthen skills.** An assortment could be used individually or all together to strengthen skills—something along the lines of a pre-externship right in the safety of your classroom.

- **Mimic clinic or physician office environment.** The contemporary case study should mimic a real clinic or physician's office and the scenarios should provide for continuous hands-on practicing of competencies.

- **Augment learning in an existing program or replace an existing program.** This grouping of case studies would be able to enhance the learning experience in any existing program or completely replace and update an existing program.

Evaluation

You might be thinking to yourself, "This sounds great but it is going to be a lot of work." Initially, it may require some additional set-up time to become familiar and organize the materials. But you won't need to write evaluations or create ways in which to grade the material: *Rubrics have been created for every case study.*

Rubric design includes:

- Identification of all main and supporting competencies
- A template for grading
- Allows for evaluation of skills in gradients
- Beginning rubrics allow for error and growth
- Later rubrics include less room for error as students advance in skill and knowledge

Before You Begin

Finally, I need to provide you with a little more background before getting started. First, the student is put into a simulation in which he or she is an employee of

Kaden Medical Clinic (read *Welcome to* Kaden Medical Clinic on page xxi). Then learn about the biographies of all of the practitioners of the clinic–these are the characters each student will work for and with (read the *Health Care Practitioner Biographies* on page xxiii). All of the forms required to complete each case study are provided on the CD-ROM that accompanies the book.

You will need to ensure that all equipment and supplies are available (although not set out). To the best of your ability, the classroom should resemble a physician's office or clinic (reception area, examination room, laboratory area, etc.). The case studies are designed to accommodate:

- Several groups of students working on the same case study

- One group doing research, answering questions, preparing correspondence or doing basic "desk" work

- One group designated as administrative medical assistants and/or clinical medical assistants (requiring peer mentoring, but not direct instructor involvement—vital signs, interviewing the patient, intake, insurance claims, etc.)

- One group requiring direct instructor (practitioner) supervision (invasive procedures)

Several case studies can be going at the same time because in a real clinic several patients would be seen at the same time. Again, the class can be broken into several groups and each group assigned a case study. Within the small groups students can then be assigned parts as written above.

If not used as an entire program, the case studies can alternately be used to supplement a current course topic. For example, if the lecture topic is "Burns," the case study on burns can be enacted after the lecture. The potential is limitless, but the difficult part has been done and now you have the time to focus on the learning.

Please enjoy using these case studies with my sincere gratitude for the opportunity to play a role in your students' education.

Kathryn A. Kalanick

About the Author

Kathryn Kalanick has been a postsecondary educator for 30 years. Before starting her own company, her last position was that of Director of Education for the Career Academy in Anchorage, Alaska. Ms. Kalanick has been instrumental in developing numerous allied health care curriculums, for both on-ground and online programs, for national accreditation. Ms. Kalanick serves as a member of several educational advisory boards nationwide and has served as a member of both the Medical Assistant and Phlebotomy Examination Review teams for NCCT and currently serves as the chair for NCCT's Board of Testing.

She currently owns and operates Educational Pathways in Utah and works as an author, consultant, invited speaker, curriculum developer, and instructional designer. She is a certified medical assistant and a nationally certified phlebotomy technician as well as one of the nation's first certified postsecondary instructors to earn the CPI (NCCT) credential.

Reviewers

Estelle Coffino, MPA, RRT, CPFT, CCMA
Program Director/Chairperson, Allied Health Programs
The College of Westchester, White Plains, NY

Sharon Harris-Pelliccia, BS, RPA
Department Chair, Medical Studies
Mildred Elley, Albany, NY

Kim Hockaday, NCMA, NCET, NCICS
Director of Medical Assisting
Carrington College, Reno, NV

Lawanna Lambert, LVN
Instructor, Externship Coordinator
American Commercial College, Odessa, TX

Penny Lee, CMA (AAMA), CAHI
Program Director of Medical Assisting
MedTech College, Greenwood, IN

Tabitha Lyons, NCMA, NRMA
Dean of Education
Anthem Institute, Parsipanny, NJ

Alice Macomber, RN, RMA, CPI, AHI, RPT, BXO
Medical Assisting Program Director
Keiser University, Port St. Lucie, FL

Barbara Marchelletta, BS, CMA(AAMA), CPC
Director, Allied Health
Beal College, Bangor, ME

Wilsetta McClain, MBA, RMA, NCICS, NR-CMA, NCPT
Department Chair
Baker College, Auburn Hills, MI

Deanna Melton-Riddle, DHA, MSA, CMA(AAMA), BA
Contributing Faculty
Walden University, Chicago, IL

Donna Otis, LPN
Medical Instructor
Metro Business College, Rolla, MO

Sandra K. Rains, MBA, RHIA
Chairperson, Health Information Technology Program
DeVry University, Columbus, OH

Adrienne Reaves, EdD
Medical Assisting Program Chair
Westwood College, Calumet City, IL

Cindy Thompson
Associate Department Chair/Program Director Allied Health
Davenport University, Saginaw, MI

Welcome to Kaden Medical Clinic

Dear Student,

As part of your training, you have been accepted as a student medical assistant and will be employed at *Kaden Medical Clinic* (KMC). KMC is a simulated clinic experience and is designed to facilitate your learning process by providing you with real-life case studies that will guide you through practicing your skill sets.

KMC has several physicians on staff. You will read about them in the *Health Care Practitioner Biographies* section on page xxiii. Their names are Dr. Carla Carlson, Dr. George Greggs, Dr. Wilhelmina Wertz, and Dr. Barry Bledsole. Your instructor(s) will assume the roles of these physicians in the simulated practice. You will also work with Chris Taylor, PA, and Bjourn Sedrickson, NP, as well as registered nurses Susah Patel and Mary Colleen Callaghan. Their biographies are also included.

As a new employee, there are a few guidelines you should become familiar with before your first day in the clinic. These guidelines are the same basic guidelines you will be expected to follow in a real medical practice and have only been adapted for KMC where absolutely necessary.

1. You will treat all patients (classmates), coworkers (classmates), and physicians (instructors) with respect, courtesy, compassion, and honesty.

2. You will, at all times while working in the clinic, adhere to the KMC dress code:

   - Student medical assistants must not deviate from the approved KMC uniform, which consists of scrubs with white socks and shoes.

   - Nails must be maintained at a clinical length without colored polish.

   - Shoulder length or longer hair must be restrained from the face.

   - One earring per ear is permitted. All other visible body piercing hardware must be removed.

   - One ring per hand is acceptable.

   - Visors and hats are not permitted.

   - Student Identification must be worn at all times.

   - Personal protective equipment (PPE) will be worn when appropriate.

3. All laboratory rules and regulations will be followed as posted and as outlined by the Occupational Safety and Health Administration (OSHA), Clinical Laboratory Improvement Amendments (CLIA), and all other applicable regulatory agencies as appropriate.

4. Confidentiality will be strictly enforced through Health Insurance Portability and Accessibility Act (HIPAA) protocol.

5. You are responsible for your own work. This includes all components of every assigned procedure, including setup and cleanup for the procedure.

6. Before starting any procedure, think the process through: Do you have all of the required equipment and supplies? Do you have the patient's chart? Do you have the physician's orders (case study)? Refer to a medical assisting textbook as a guideline for performing specific procedure steps. If you are unsure on how to perform a procedure or have questions regarding one, ask the physician (instructor) before starting. This will help you increase your critical thinking skills. Of course, if you have questions during a procedure never hesitate to ask your instructor for help and guidance.

7. Every procedure will be properly documented as outlined in our *Documentation Policies and Procedures* (see page xxv). Documentation procedures and techniques will be frequently audited by classmates and instructors. Any procedure that is not properly documented will not be considered performed.

8. For any medications that are ordered, you will need to document the number and amount of medications given and the route and site of administration as well as the name of the medication, lot number, and expiration date in the patient's medical record. Show your calculations on a separate sheet of paper. (See *Documentation Policies and Procedures*, page xxv.)

9. When documenting a procedure, use the actual date and time. In parentheses next to the patient name, write the name of the student with whom you worked in completing the case study (that is the person on whom you took the vital signs, from whom you drew the blood, to whom you gave the injection, etc.).

10. *Remember: All patient documentation is considered legal documentation and can be used in a court of law so be concise and complete.*

We would like to welcome you on board as part of our medical team. We look forward to working with you and it is our sincere hope that this is an outstanding learning experience for everyone involved.

Kaden Medical Clinic Administration

Health Care Practitioner Biographies

Dr. Carla Carlson was a retired family practice physician. She is a 1966 graduate of the University of Washington School of Medicine. She practiced medicine in the Spokane area for 20 years within a multidoctor practice, where she specialized in women's health issues. She sits on the advisory boards of the University of Washington and Planned Parenthood. She is the immediate past president of the Washington State Medical Society. When presented with the opportunity to join the KMC staff in 2002, she abandoned all thoughts of retirement. Dr. Carlson likes everything neat and tidy. She is full of energy and always on the go and she expects her medical assistants to be the same.

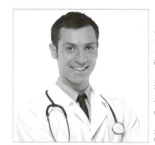

Dr. George Greggs has the distinction of being the youngest medical practitioner in Arizona history. He graduated from the University of Arizona at the age of 19 and went on to medical school and graduated at the age of 22. He was the medical director for a prominent internal medicine practice with 13 practitioners on staff. He joined the KMC family last year at the age of 35. Dr. Greggs is all business—he is a very dedicated physician and likes to stay current with the most sophisticated and up-to-date technology. He expects his medical assistants to stay current in all of the latest trends, techniques, and procedures. He requires his medical assistants to do their own research if they have a question. Once they have formulated an answer, he is then more than happy to discuss and elaborate. He particularly is impressed with his medical assistants who can critically think through a situation and has been known to give bonuses and incentives to medical assistants who excel in this area.

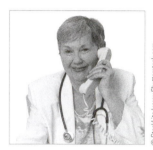

Dr. Wilhelmina Wertz started her distinguished career as a medical assistant in 1976. In 1978, she became a paramedic with the Denver Fire Department. After running on the ambulance for three years Dr. Wertz decided that she wanted more. She returned to school and became a well-respected surgeon in Maryland. Dr. Wertz was instrumental in perfecting the design and function of the most favored pacemaker in use for cardiac patients. Dr. Wertz, having been a medical assistant, is very proactive in promoting the profession and she lets her medical assistants do whatever they show an interest and ability to do. She likes to teach, but you must be prepared and show initiative. Dr. Wertz has no tolerance for slackers; however, if you want to learn or try something new, she will guide you through every step of the way. Dr. Wertz has been a welcome addition to the KMC staff for the past three years.

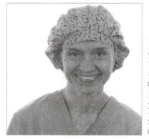

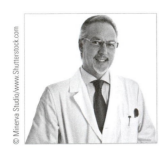

Dr. Barry Bledsole is known around KMC for his great sense of humor and practical jokes. Dr. Bledsole brings a refreshing view of medicine to the clinic and his patients adore him. He was an army doctor in Vietnam in the late 1960s, and after two tours of duty he settled into the emergency room at Houston General where he ran the night shift with precision. He is best known for his bedside manner because he has the skill in making every patient feel, regardless of social status or condition, as if that patient is the most important patient he has ever seen. He joined the staff at KMC five years ago.

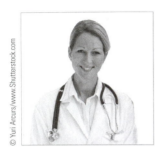

Chris Taylor, PA, has worked for KMC for six months. She is an excellent diagnostician and is held in high esteem with the physicians. Chris primarily works with Dr. Bledsole and considers him her greatest mentor. Their philosophies and sense of humor blend perfectly. Chris is outgoing, friendly, and easy to talk to. Most of the registered nurses (RNs) and medical assistants on staff at KMC go to Chris with their questions. She always makes time to respond and educate.

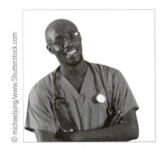

Bjourn Sedrickson, NP, is a new hire at KMC. He has worked as an RN for 12 years, most notably at the Huntsman Cancer Institute in Salt Lake City, Utah, as a surgical nurse, and he is very honored to be asked to join the KMC staff. As a new nurse practitioner, Bjourn is looking forward to bringing his experience from working with patients with cancer to the clinic.

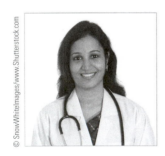

Susah Patel and Mary Colleen Callaghan are both RNs who work for KMC. Susah has been an RN for 4 years, and Mary Colleen has been an RN for 22 years. Both are very supportive of the medical assistant profession and understand the role that medical assistants play in the workforce. They are both very willing to answer questions and encourage the medical assistants on staff to perform to the highest level of their scope of practice. However, a medical assistant who oversteps his or her bounds will quickly find either Susah or Mary Colleen reeling him or her back in with a quick reprimand.

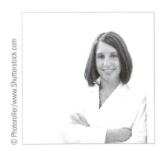

Documentation Policies and Procedures

When documenting in the patient's medical record, it is important to remember the following:

1. Complete all documentation in black ink. Any item written in any other color of ink will not be considered documented.

2. Use medical abbreviations and medical terminology in charting when appropriate. Any documentation that contains medical terms or abbreviations not correctly spelled or used will be considered incorrect and will not be accepted as proof of documentation. Look up medical terms and abbreviations when in doubt.

3. Use the patient's exact words when describing the symptoms.

4. If you cannot remember the exact words, it is okay to use medical terms that mean the same thing. Just be sure to record everything that the patient reports to you.

5. Document any patient teaching that you do with the patient and/or significant other (family, friend, etc.). Examples of documentation are included in Table FM-3.

TABLE FM-3   Examples of Patient Education Documentation

Instructed in technique for daily sterile dressing change. Able to return demo without difficulty.
Patient and spouse instructed in use of blood glucose meter. Return demo by patient and spouse with minimal prompting. Patient states patient will obtain additional strips to go with meter provided from office. Aware that insurance may or may not pay for strips. Instructed to check BG qid and record in BG record book. Instructed to return with BG record book in one week for appointment with Dr. Carlson.

© Cengage Learning 2013

6. The assumption is that you are talking about the patient unless you indicate otherwise in your documentation.

7. Always date and time all documentation with the date and time it is being written.

8. Appropriately sign, with first initial and full last name and the credential "Student Medical Assistant" (SMA), all documentation, and eliminate any blank spaces at the end of each line (Table FM-4).

TABLE FM-4   Example of Signing Documentation

R. McKinley, SMA ---

© Cengage Learning 2013

9. Document as soon as the procedure is completed so nothing is forgotten.

10. ***DO NOT*** prechart.

11. When charting medications, include the following:

    a. Name of drug

    b. Dose given (remember to write a zero before the dosage amount if less than 1 mL. Example: 0.5 mL)

    c. Route (Oral, Topical, Parenteral)

    d. Location (IM, ID, or SubQ)

    e. Lot number in case there is a recall of the medication

    f. Expiration date

    g. Note whether or not there was any reaction and how patient tolerated the procedure

    h. Record any follow-up visits and results for immunizations (e.g., PPD reading in 48–72 hours)

12. Include a note in the patient's chart whenever you speak with the patient on the telephone. Include the contents of the conversation and the outcome. Table FM-5 provides several examples.

TABLE FM-5   Examples of Documenting Telephone Calls

Pt. called for a refill of Synthroid, 125 mcg, po, q day. Phoned to Corner Rx at 1515 hrs.
Pt. called for refill of Darvocet-N, 100 mg, po, q 6 hr prn. Told patient we cannot refill over the phone. Patient asked to talk to Dr. Bledsole personally. Offered to make an appointment. Pt refused and insisted on talking with Dr. Bledsole on the phone first. Note left for Dr. Bledsole.
Ms. Smith (patient's mother) called that Johnny has a runny nose, cough, and fever. Wants to know if it is okay to give liquid Tylenol. Spoke with Dr. Greggs. Dr. Greggs gave okay for liquid Tylenol, ½ tsp, po, q4h, prn fever over 101 degrees F. Ms. Smith verbally repeated instructions for Tylenol. Instructed to bring Johnny in if symptoms worsen or are not better in 7 days.

© Cengage Learning 2013

13. Document any procedure administered to a patient. Table FM-6 provides several examples.

TABLE FM-6   Examples of Documenting Procedures

Strep test ordered and completed with negative (positive) results.
Hemoccult cards ×3 given to patient with instructions to return them to the office tomorrow morning. Patient instructions given for procedure. Make sure results are then written in the patient's chart and reviewed by physician.
ECG performed per physician's order. *(Remember that you are not authorized to read the ECG. It should be reviewed by the physician, if abnormal, before letting the patient leave.)*
UA dip performed. Lab slip attached.
CBC, Lipids, and CMP drawn from left arm, antecubital area, and no difficulties noted.

© Cengage Learning 2013

14. Document all outpatient or inpatient hospital stays or procedures.

15. Use a single line through incorrect documentation. Be sure to ***initial and date*** above the line. Proceed with correct documentation.
    Remember: If it isn't documented, it didn't happen. When in doubt, write it out.

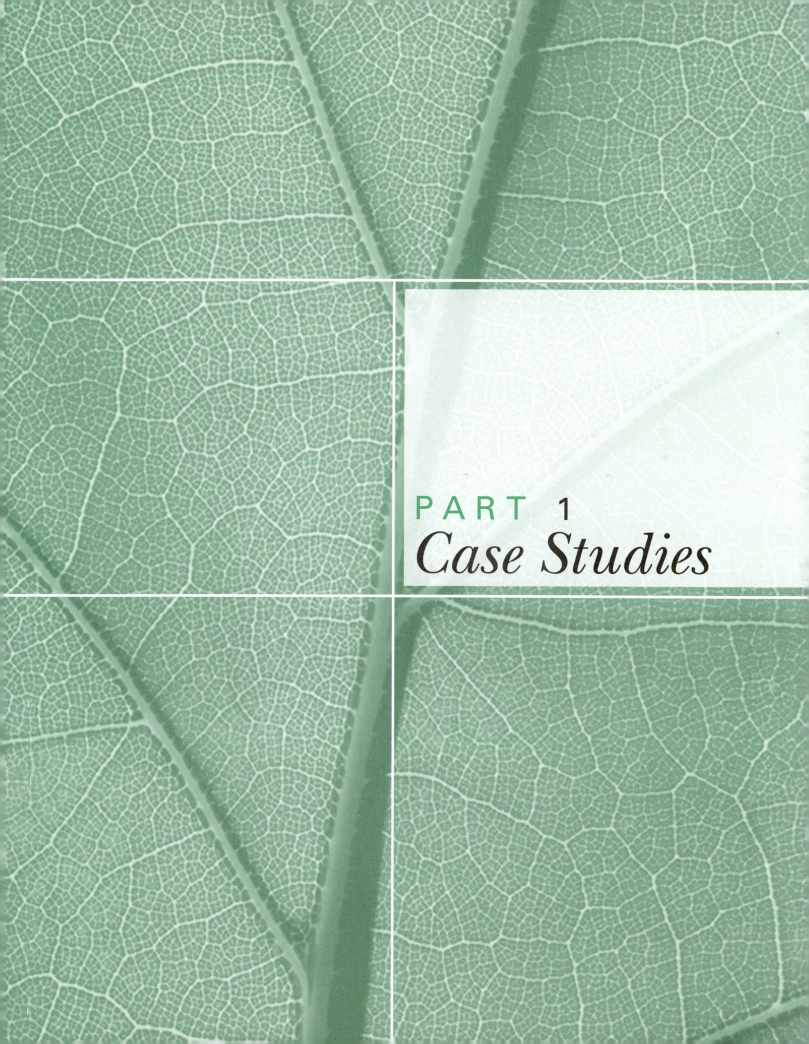

PART 1
Case Studies

CASE STUDY 1

Medical Assistant Responsibilities

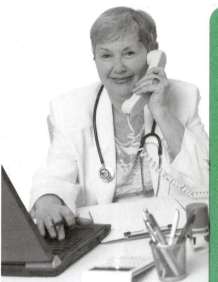

ADMINISTRATIVE

With the recent termination of a medical assistant at KMC, Dr. Carlson is short staffed. Until Dr. Carlson can hire a replacement, you and one other medical assistant must share administrative and clinical responsibilities. Before you leave for the day, Dr. Carlson has asked you and the other medical assistant to meet to create a plan on how you will distribute the responsibilities and to e-mail her a detailed outline of the distribution. She has also asked that you both make sure that the reception area and examination rooms are ready for the day. There are 11 patients on Dr. Carlson's schedule for tomorrow and she does not want you to cancel any appointments. She has approved three hours of overtime pay for each of you. Make suitable arrangements in your personal lives to accommodate staying late to work. When you discover who the other medical assistant is, you inwardly groan. You do not care for this person and have had disagreements with this person in the past. You must maintain a professional attitude and communicate in a professional manner with tact, diplomacy, courtesy, and personal integrity. Remember: Competent patient care is the goal.

Respond to the following questions and perform the listed skills. *Skills will be accomplished by pairing with a classmate. Your instructor will assign you a partner to complete this case study. You may not change partners. Role-play the case study where indicated.*

1. With your partner, create a general list of the responsibilities that will need to be covered tomorrow. Divide the list into administrative and clinical responsibilities. You must both agree to an item before placing it on the list.

2. Assign each responsibility to one of you. Again you must agree. You may not assign all administrative tasks to one person and all clinical tasks to the other person, nor can you divide the day with one partner being the administrative assistant in the morning and the clinical assistant in the afternoon. Be conscious of workflow and time management.

3. Prioritize the list by assigning a number value to each item with a number (1) identifying high-priority items—must be completed; a number (2) identifying midlevel priorities—should be completed; and a number (3) identifying low-level priorities—would be nice to complete tomorrow.

4. In a word processing document key your list of duties, divided by administrative and clinical responsibilities in order of priority. Identify which one of you will be handling each responsibility. E-mail the document to Dr. Carlson (your instructor).

5. Create an appointment schedule for tomorrow with 11 patients, using the modified wave scheduling protocol. Print a copy for Dr. Carlson. (Submit it to your instructor.) Names and reasons to be seen will be fictitious, but the length of appointment times assigned must be realistic.

6. Your instructor will determine whether this step will be accomplished physically or in writing. Prepare the reception area and two examination rooms. If this step will be accomplished physically, you and your partner should share equally in the responsibilities. Your instructor will inspect your work. If it is determined that this step will be accomplished in writing, personally describe what elements are involved in preparing the reception area and two examination rooms. Submit a hardcopy to your instructor.

7. Describe in writing what accommodations you would personally need to make in order to work three hours late. Print one copy and then use KMC's photocopier to make one copy, enlarged to 125%. (This step should be completed individually.) Submit it to your instructor.

8. Describe in writing any conflicts that you and the "other medical assistant" role-played or that you and your partner actually faced and the outcome. If no conflict occurred, acknowledge this and describe areas of conflict that may have occurred given another partner or coworker. (This step should be completed individually.) Submit the document to your instructor via the delivery method requested.

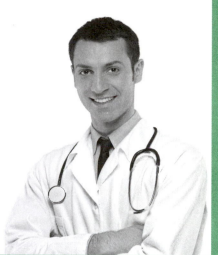

© Ljupco Smokovski/www.shutterstock.com

ADMINISTRATIVE

CASE STUDY **2**

Administrative Duties and Telephone Techniques–Day 1

Susan, the administrative assistant who runs the front office, will be out sick for at least two days. Dr. Greggs has asked you to fill in for her. Susan is responsible for fielding telephone calls, taking messages, scheduling appointments, and making reminder calls.

Respond to the following questions and perform the listed skills. *Skills will be accomplished by pairing with a classmate. Role-play the case study where indicated. Respond to the following telephone calls by role-playing with a small group of students. Rotate positions until everyone in your group has been the medical assistant and has answered each call.*

1. KMC accepts telephone calls between 9:00 and 10:30 a.m. from patients seeking appointment slots that may be available for the day. It is 9:20 a.m. now and the call volume is exceedingly large. You are responsible for five telephone lines; three have patients currently holding on the line to speak with you and the other two are ringing. The clinic would like you to answer the telephones, if possible, before the fourth ring to verify that there are no patients with emergencies or other physician offices calling. Study the following before role-playing this scenario.

   a. Be sure to professionally answer the telephone. What is the correct way to answer the telephone in this situation?

   _____

   _____

   _____

   _____

   b. Demonstrate effective screening of all telephone calls to determine the nature of the call.

   c. Answer at least five calls during your role-play.

2. It is 9:30 a.m. and you have three patients on hold. You are currently speaking to a patient who is experiencing "a tingling feeling all over" and her "mind feels cloudy and confused." You have determined that two of the callers on hold are patients seeking appointments with Dr. Greggs and the other caller is requesting to speak with Dr. Bledsole about some laboratory results. Study the following before role-playing this scenario.

   a. How would you respond to the patient currently on the telephone with you? Should you gather more information from her? If so, what type of information?

   _____

   _____

   _____

   _____

   b. Does she need an emergency appointment at the clinic or should she be referred to the emergency room? (Your response will be based on the answers to your questions through role-play.) Include your thoughts and answers to these questions in your role-play.

   c. After checking the physician schedule, you return to the caller who is requesting to speak to Dr. Bledsole and inform him that the physician is not in until 1:00 p.m. The patient would like to leave a message for Dr. Bledsole. What type of information should you ask the patient when taking a message? Take the message and submit it to Dr. Bledsole for evaluation.

   _____

   _____

   _____

   _____

   d. There is only one available appointment left for the day with Dr. Greggs. How do you determine which patient should be scheduled today with Dr. Greggs? Should you schedule one of the patients with another physician? Be sure to appropriately schedule the appointments and end the call.

   _____

   _____

   _____

   _____

CASE STUDY **3**

Administrative Duties and Telephone Techniques–Day 2

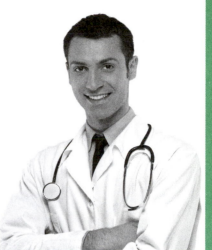

Susan, the administrative assistant who runs the front office, will be out sick for at least two days. Dr. Greggs has asked you to fill in for her. Susan is responsible for fielding telephone calls, taking messages, scheduling appointments, and making reminder calls.

Respond to the following questions and perform the listed skills. *Skills will be accomplished by pairing with a classmate. Role-play the case study where indicated. Respond to the following telephone calls by role-playing with a small group of students. Rotate positions until everyone in your group has been the medical assistant and has answered each call.*

1. Someone from the hospital laboratory is on the telephone and is requesting to speak with Chris Taylor, PA. You transfer the call to Chris. However, a minute later you answer the telephone and it is the caller from the hospital laboratory requesting to speak with Chris again (the call was transferred to her voice mail box). The caller informs you that Chris has requested some laboratory work be performed stat and is following through with her request to telephone the results before sending them. Study the following before role-playing this scenario.

   a. You search for Chris and find that she is in an examination room with a patient. What is the appropriate course of action in this situation?

   _____

   _____

   _____

   _____

   b. If you decide to interrupt Chris, how would you maintain confidentiality and professional tact and courtesy while informing her that someone from the laboratory is on the telephone regarding her stat request for a patient?

   _____

   _____

   _____

   _____

2. After Chris receives the results from the laboratory, she requests that you call the patient and schedule a follow-up appointment with Chris within the next two days. You call the patient and he begs you to tell him the results of his tests. You explain to the patient that you cannot tell him the results and that Chris would like him to come in to see her. The patient apologizes and schedules an appointment.

   a. Schedule the appointment and maintain professional tact, courtesy, and communication during this situation.

   b. What are the legal and professional ramifications of informing a patient of his or her laboratory results? Research and write a one-page report of your findings. Submit the report to your instructor.

3. It is 3:00 p.m. and it is time to make reminder calls to the patients who are on tomorrow's schedule. You are on your last telephone call and the patient is elderly and hard of hearing. After a lengthy amount of time trying to communicate the reminder to the patient, you find that she will not be able to keep her scheduled appointment. Study the following before role-playing this scenario.

   a. Keep in mind that there are still patients in the waiting area and they may be able to overhear your conversation with the patient. How do you maintain patient confidentiality while responding to this telephone call?

   _____

   _____

   _____

   _____

   b. How will you overcome this communication difficulty with this patient? In what ways do you need to adapt your communication style to be sure that the patient understands what you are saying to her?

   _____

   _____

   _____

   _____

   c. How would you go about rescheduling her appointment? With the communication barrier, would you opt to schedule her appointment in a week or more so that you can mail her an appointment card before her appointment? Is it ethical to locate a next of kin or emergency number in her file so that you can reschedule her appointment? Research this situation and answer the questions in a one-page written report.

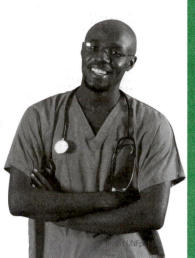

CASE STUDY **4**

Body Divisions, Planes, Positions, Draping/ Gowning, and Ethics

ADMINISTRATIVE

Some of the staff have been explaining gowning and positioning to patients incorrectly and in an inappropriate manner. Bjourn Sedrickson is concerned that some of the staff may need a refresher course in body divisions, planes, positions, draping, and ethics. He has asked you to prepare and present a refresher course for the staff meeting next week.

Respond to the following questions and perform the refresher course as ordered by Bjourn. *Skills will be accomplished by pairing with a classmate. Role-play the case study where indicated.*

1. Prepare a 10-minute refresher course as outlined above. The course should contain the following components:

   - Written presentation (document resources).

   - Visual presentation (examples may include posters, PowerPoint presentation, physical demonstration, or any combination).

   - Professional communication should be addressed. For example, the descriptive procedures should adhere to appropriate terminology.

   - Sections on body divisions, planes, positions, draping, and ethics should be included, along with patient vulnerability, possible sexual harassment, and liability of improper conduct.

   - Demonstration of how to display a professional attitude.

2. Oral presentation: Conduct your 10-minute refresher course to a minimum of five classmates. Your instructor may request presentations to be given to the entire class.

3. Your instructor may assign you to work on this project in small groups.

4. Submit the presentation to Bjourn Sedrickson in writing to be added to the office policy and procedures manual.

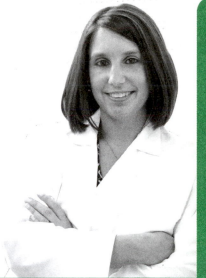

ADMINISTRATIVE

CASE STUDY 5

Filing–Medical Records

Marcy is going to complete her externship at KMC. Mary Colleen Callaghan has asked you to monitor Marcy's work and to provide her with the opportunity to accomplish tasks in the various areas required by her school. She would like for you to begin Marcy's externship in the administrative setting. You decide that the first thing that Marcy should experience is how to file and maintain records.

Respond to the following questions and perform the listed skills. *Skills will be accomplished by pairing with a classmate. Role-play the case study where indicated.*

1. Research, as needed, and then have a clear idea of how you will present this information to Marcy. Role-play the scenario, covering the following topics:

   - Basic filing systems

   - Special filing systems

   - Filing guidelines (storing, protecting/safekeeping, transferring)

   - Organization of the patient medical record

   - Types of medical records (problem- or source-oriented)

   - Collecting information for medical records

   - Making corrections in a medical record

   - Retaining and purging of medical records

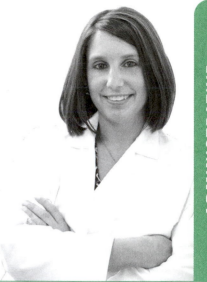

© Photoroller/www.Shutterstock.com

ADMINISTRATIVE

CASE STUDY **6**

Equipment Supply and Inventory

Marcy has mastered the filing and maintaining of records (from Case Study 5) and is ready for her next assignment. It is time for the monthly inventory of supplies in both the administrative and clinical aspects of the clinic. You decide to teach Marcy how to correctly inventory and order supplies. KMC maintains an inventory of supplies that are estimated to last one month.

Marcy, under your supervision, will be required to verify that all supplies are up to date, in stock, and essential. One of the clinic's suppliers has raised prices for products and shipping to an unreasonable amount. Ask Marcy to research costs and suppliers for the clinical supplies that are needed and to report her findings to you. Also, the clinic's electrocardiograph (ECG) has finally worn out. You will need to locate a manufacturer and the cost of a new machine.

Marcy has reported her findings and you find them to be reasonable and cost effective. You will order the clinical supplies together via fax, providing a teaching moment for Marcy. Marcy will then be prepared to place the administrative supply order next week.

Respond to the following questions and perform the listed skills. *Skills will be accomplished by pairing with a classmate. Role-play the case study where indicated.*

1. With a partner, inventory all clinical supplies located in KMC's (your classroom's) laboratory. Provide the completed list to your instructor. (Note: Your instructor may only assign a certain portion of the laboratory supplies.)

2. Locate at least two vendors and research the costs for the following clinical products:

   - 20 × 36 pediatric gowns

   - 40 × 60 drape sheets

   - 2 × 2 gauze sponges

   - Reagent test strips (10 parameters)

   - Pipettes

- Pregnancy tests
- Examination table paper
- EDTA Vacutainer tubes
- Disposable, nonlatex, powder-free gloves (sizes small, medium, and large)
- Pediatric lancets
- Kelly forceps
- Computerized ECG machine (new)

3. Prepare an itemized list and submit it to Mary Colleen Callaghan.

4. Role-play placing the order via a fax. Call to confirm that the fax arrived.

CASE STUDY 7

Administrative Duties and Training

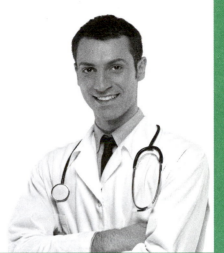

© Ljupco Smokovski/www.Shutterstock.com

Susan is still sick and will be out for the rest of the week. Dr. Greggs has hired a temporary medical assistant, named Jake, because you are needed for your normal duties. However, you must teach Jake about the type of scheduling that each physician prefers and how to manage and follow the protocol for answering the telephone, taking messages, and confirming appointments.

Respond to the following questions and perform the listed skills. *Skills will be accomplished by pairing with a classmate. Role-play the case study where indicated.*

1. Familiarize Jake with KMC's protocols for answering the telephone, taking messages, confirming appointments, and scheduling patients.

2. Demonstrate to Jake how to matrix the appointment book (this may be through practice management software or a hardcopy of one week's schedule, as indicated by your instructor).

3. Observe Jake, through role-play, answering the telephone and scheduling a new patient. Provide Jake with constructive criticism for improving his skills. Remember: The goal of "training" Jake for this temporary position is to free you up to work your normal duties. You are responsible for his training and will be held accountable should errors occur.

CASE STUDY **8**

Processing Incoming Mail and Posting Payments

The mail has just been delivered to the clinic and needs to be processed. You have received the following pieces of mail:

1. Thank-you card from Samantha Gunner for the care and kindness that the office staff and Dr. Carlson gave to her grandmother during her treatment for breast cancer.

2. Waiting room copies of three magazines.

3. Letter marked "Personal" to Dr. Greggs. Invitation to present at a symposium next month in Denver, Colorado.

4. Payment from James Fowler (personal amount due from his visit regarding his hypertension). He paid $175 on his $360 bill.

5. Medicare update.

6. Monthly report from ABC Collection Agency on outstanding accounts:

   • Stan Torrey—Account uncollectible. Patient incarcerated. Write off $345.

   • Adeline Blackett—Collected $200 on balance of $4,365.56. Payment arrangements made at $200 per month until paid in full. Check for $200 included.

   • Jamie Henderson—No contact made.

   • Noella Winderland—$25 payment on balance of $350. Check for $23 included ($2 of the payment as fee to the collection agency).

7. Payment from Veronica Staples (personal amount due from her Pap and breast examinations). She paid $46 on her account, bringing the balance to zero.

8. Promotional material for a new cardiac instrument addressed to Dr. Wertz.

9. Monthly bank statement for KMC.

10. Covington Insurance, malpractice insurance statement, payment of $15,780.49 due in 10 days.

11. Crabapple Investment, LLC, lease statement, payment of $8,793 due in 15 days.

12. Concorde Corporation, utility statement, payment of $1,322.54 due in 10 days.

13. DataMaster, telephone and Internet service statement, payment of $596.81 due in 21 days.

14. Flyer requesting donation to local Little League team for uniforms.

15. Community newsletter from the chamber of commerce.

Respond to the following questions and perform the listed skills.

1. Prioritize the mail you received today. Describe in writing how each piece of mail will be processed and dispatched.

_____

_____

_____

_____

2. Accurately post payments and update patient accounts. Your instructor will inform you of how to proceed on posting payments to accounts, either electronically or manually.

CASE STUDY **9**

Research for Presentation

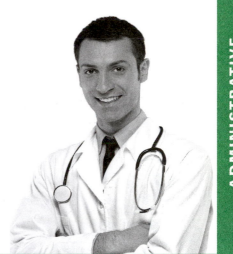

ADMINISTRATIVE

Dr. Greggs has been asked to write an article for the *Journal of the American Medical Association (JAMA)* on the topic of prostate cancer and the use of antioxidants. He must submit the article in two weeks. He has asked you to do some preliminary research for him. He suggests that you do an Internet search using the keywords *prostate cancer* and *antioxidants.* He would like for you to pull any information you can locate that is relevant for the past 12 months. He would then like you to compile a list of Web sites that he can use as a point of reference for writing his article. He is especially interested in any reports or studies that have been done by other physicians. He would also like for you to obtain contact information—telephone numbers, e-mail addresses, and so on—for the authoring physicians of the studies so he can contact them for interviews. He would then like for you to write a 500-word report either supporting or denying the effectiveness of the use of antioxidants in treating prostate cancer, citing which article(s) you used to draw your conclusions.

Respond to the following questions and perform the listed skills.

1. Search the Internet for related articles using the keywords *prostate cancer* and *antioxidants.* Locate at least two reports or studies that have been written or conducted by physicians. Articles should be dated within the past 12 months.

2. Locate and provide at least three sources of contact information for physician(s) authoring reports or studies. Contact information can include a telephone number, an e-mail address, or a physical address that Dr. Greggs can use to interview the physicians.

3. Write a 500-word report either supporting or denying the effectiveness of the use of antioxidants in treating prostate cancer, using either MLA or APA format (as directed by your instructor). Cite the article(s) used to support your view.

   a. Submit a first draft of your report via e-mail (your instructor will provide you with an e-mail address to submit your report) to Dr. Greggs (your instructor). Dr. Greggs will make any corrections he deems necessary and will return a hardcopy to you, using appropriate proofreader's marks. You will then make corrections and submit a final draft of your report via e-mail to Dr. Greggs.

b. Both the first draft and final draft of your report will be graded on content, correct use of medical terminology, sentence structure, grammar, and punctuation.

CASE STUDY **10**

Banking Procedures and Preparing Outgoing Mail

The following mail has been processed and the payments have been posted to patient accounts. You now have the responsibility to prepare the checks for the payments that are due, preparing the received payments for deposit, and reconciling the bank statement.

- Payment from James Fowler (personal amount due from his visit regarding his hypertension). He paid $175 on his $360 bill.

- Monthly report from ABC Collection Agency on outstanding accounts:

    o Stan Torrey—Account uncollectible. Patient incarcerated. Write off $345.

    o Adeline Blackett—Collected $200 on balance of $4,365.56. Payment arrangements made at $200 per month until paid in full. Check for $200 included.

    o Jamie Henderson—No contact made.

    o Noella Winderland—$25 payment on balance of $350. Check for $23 included ($2 of the payment as fee to the collection agency).

- Payment from Veronica Staples (personal amount due from her Pap and breast examinations). She paid $46 on her account, bringing the balance to zero.

- Monthly bank statement for KMC.

- Covington Insurance, malpractice insurance statement, payment of $15,780.49 due in 10 days.

- Crabapple Investment, LLC, lease statement, payment of $8,793 due in 15 days.

- Concorde Corporation, utility statement, payment of $1,322.54 due in 10 days.

- DataMaster, telephone and Internet service statement, payment of $596.81 due in 21 days.

Respond to the following questions and perform the listed skills.

1. Prepare the checks for all payments due for the month (use today's date).
2. Prepare the payments due for outgoing mail.
3. Prepare a bank deposit for today's receivables (use today's date).
4. Reconcile the bank statement.

CASE STUDY **11**

Follow-Up Appointments

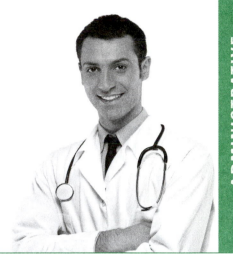

During Gideon Straus's sigmoidoscopy, Dr. Greggs discovered three small, flat polyps. Dr. Greggs removed the polyps and sent them to be tested for cancer. The polyps were cancerous. Mr. Straus underwent radiation and chemotherapy treatments for six weeks with some success. It was decided, however, to remove a section of Mr. Straus's bowel and perform an ileostomy. Mr. Straus may have the ileostomy reversed in the future.

You scheduled Mr. Straus for a follow-up appointment with Dr. Greggs in one week. You telephoned Mr. Straus before his appointment to remind him of the scheduled time. On the day of the appointment, he arrives right on schedule. Dr. Greggs would like you to do a patient interview, asking pertinent questions to determine the quality of Gideon's health since the surgery.

Respond to the following questions and perform the listed skills as ordered by Dr. Greggs. *Skills will be accomplished by pairing with a classmate. Role-play the case study where indicated.*

1. Role-play a reminder telephone call to Mr. Straus.

2. Before your interaction with Mr. Straus, research standard postsurgical instructions and formulate at least 10 questions to be asked during your "interview" with Gideon. The questions should be in regard to his post-op health, lingering effects (such as pain), and any concerns that Gideon may be having. You should develop exploratory, open-ended, and direct questions that, when asked in a professional and caring manner, would elicit an informative answer.

3. "Interview" Mr. Straus and document his responses in his file. Be sure to focus on your interviewing techniques and your ability to observe, actively listen, and provide appropriate feedback.

4. Dr. Greggs has requested that you post your list of questions to the policy and procedure manual after he reviews them. Submit your list of questions in writing to Dr. Greggs.

5. Schedule a follow-up appointment for Mr. Straus in six weeks and provide him with an appointment reminder card.

CASE STUDY **12**

Community Outreach Interview

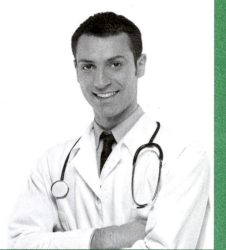

ADMINISTRATIVE

Cassie Garrett is a high school student who lives next door to Dr. Greggs. She has asked him if someone at his office would be available for an interview. Cassie is writing a report titled *Microbiology: Pathogens that Influence Disease Processes* and her teacher requires that an interview be among her sources. Dr. Greggs has asked you to do the interview with Cassie when she arrives at the clinic this afternoon.

Respond to the following questions and perform the listed skills. *Skills will be accomplished by pairing with a classmate. Role-play the case study where indicated.*

1. Role-play the interview with Cassie. (Research the topic before the interview as needed.)

2. Cassie asks the following:

   • Can you define microbiology and describe how it impacts KMC?

   • Can you identify and describe the five main pathogens?

   • Can you provide an example of each pathogen as it pertains to the disease process that you see in the clinic?

   • What is Gram staining? Which pathogen is it used with? What do gram-negative and gram-positive mean? Can you provide me with an example of a disease process for each?

3. Provide to Dr. Greggs a brief overview of your responses to Cassie's questions.

CASE STUDY **13**

Ordering Administrative Equipment and Supplies

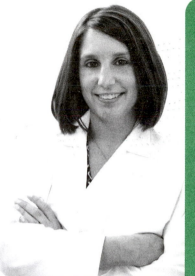

Last week, Marcy, under your supervision, completed an inventory of the clinical supplies, researched suppliers and cost, and ordered clinical supplies. You assign Marcy the task of completing an administrative inventory and formulating a list of needed items. You explain that she is to present you with this list for approval, after which she will place the order via the telephone.

Respond to the following questions and perform the listed skills. *Skills will be accomplished by pairing with a classmate. Role-play the case study where indicated.*

1. With a partner, create an inventory list of possible administrative supplies that may be located in KMC's administrative office. Provide the completed list to your instructor. (Note: Limit the list to 30 items.)

2. Locate at least two vendors and research the cost for the items on your list.

3. Prepare a typewritten itemized list, including the cost of the supplies, and submit it to Mary Colleen Callaghan, RN.

4. Role-play placing the order via telephone.

CASE STUDY **14**

Consent for Release of Medical Records

Adam Hutchins arrived at the clinic a few hours ago suffering from prescription medication withdrawal. He was transferred to the emergency room after having a seizure in your office. You just received notice from the hospital that Adam has been transferred to the psychiatric ward for observation before being transferred to a substance abuse facility.

A representative from a substance abuse facility has telephoned the clinic requesting Adam's medical record so that they may commence treatment when he arrives tomorrow. You explain that you have not received notification of consent and that you are unable to send the representative any portion of the medical record before receiving consent. You further explain that you will send the required consent form via fax.

Respond to the following questions and perform the listed skills. *Skills will be accomplished by pairing with a classmate. Role-play the case study where indicated.*

1. Role-play the telephone conversation with the representative from the substance abuse facility.

2. How will you obtain Adam's consent when he is in the psychiatric ward at the hospital? Explain in writing the need for consent in order to release medical records. Are there any HIPAA considerations involved? Defend your answer.

   _____

   _____

   _____

   _____

3. Role-play telephoning a representative from the psychiatric ward of the hospital to inform him or her of the need to obtain consent before sending Adam's medical record to the substance abuse facility.

4. Complete a consent form for release of medical records. Complete the information required and obtain Adam's signature via fax for consent to release his medical record pertaining only to information and treatment surrounding his substance abuse. (Role-play using your school's fax machine.)

5. Once you have received a legally signed consent form from Adam, copy and prepare the necessary portion of Adam's medical record to be sent (next-day service) to the substance abuse facility. The envelope should be prepared with the following address: Atwood Substance Abuse Facility, 130 Bellmont Dr., Eagle River, Alaska 99577.

CASE STUDY 15

Communication with a Distraught Patient

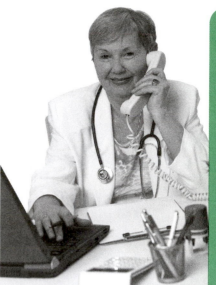

ADMINISTRATIVE

Rain Story has just called KMC to schedule an appointment with Dr. Carlson because she has heard "great things about her." Ms. Story has not been seen at the clinic before. When questioning her reason for wanting to see the physician, she states that she miscarried a year ago when she was 12 weeks pregnant and that she is now about 5 weeks pregnant. She is very nervous and would like to see Dr. Carlson as soon as possible. The next available appointment for a new patient is in a month. As you are explaining this to Rain, she begins to cry. She has heard that "Dr. Carlson is the best" and then goes on to explain to you that she is experiencing "other distressing symptoms." You agree to speak with Dr. Carlson about the situation and inform Ms. Story that you will get back with her as soon as possible.

Dr. Carlson agrees that Ms. Story needs to be seen sooner and has agreed to stay late on Wednesday next week. (However, if you are convinced and you convince Dr. Carlson that Ms. Story needs an emergency appointment, one may be set for today. This is at your instructor's discretion.) Dr. Carlson would also like you to put Ms. Rain on the cancellation list in case something comes up sooner.

Respond to the following questions and perform the listed skills as ordered by Dr. Carlson. *Skills will be accomplished by pairing with a classmate. Role-play the case study where indicated.*

1. Role-play this scenario, beginning with answering the phone. Include the appropriate techniques for answering the telephone and identifying yourself, the office, and the patient.

2. Role-play with a classmate the conversation between yourself (the medical assistant) and Ms. Story. Ms. Story may ad lib her lines to indicate a distraught patient. Indicate in writing any change of communication style that you may experience or implement to appropriately handle a distraught patient. Also, indicate the type of communication skills/techniques that you would need to exhibit in order to gather information and to ensure that Ms. Story feels comfortable speaking with you. Submit at least three grammatically correct paragraphs to your instructor for evaluation.

3. Speak with Dr. Carlson (your instructor). Dr. Carlson may or may not grant an immediate appointment depending on your appropriate presentation of the situation.

4. Place Ms. Story on the cancellation list and schedule an appointment for next Wednesday. Explain to Ms. Story that you will notify her if an appointment becomes available sooner than Wednesday next week.

5. If Dr. Carlson grants an emergency appointment as indicated in step 3, role-play the conversation between you and Ms. Story. (Note: If your instructor determines that Ms. Story must be seen today, refer to Case Study 59. Otherwise, refer to Case Study 59 at the appropriate time.)

CASE STUDY 16

Third-Party Billing and Coding

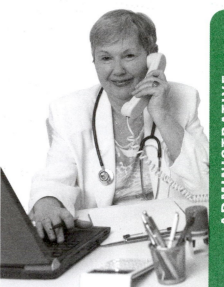

ADMINISTRATIVE

You have received and processed the mail for the day. The clinic was sent two insurance claims that were denied payment. After reviewing these two claims, you realize that the first claim for Rain Story was denied due to improper sequence of billing and that the second claim for Stacy Ardell was denied due to a coding error and the request for further information.

The first patient file to research is Rain Story. Ms. Story, a new patient, was seen at the clinic due to issues with her current pregnancy (she miscarried last year). A pregnancy test was performed to confirm pregnancy and a full urinalysis was performed as well. She was given a prenatal examination and the following blood tests were ordered and drawn: CBC, hCG, and because Dr. Carlson suspected hypothyroidism, a TSH was also ordered. Ms. Story has primary insurance coverage through Blue Cross/Blue Shield (BC/BS) and secondary coverage through Medicaid.

The second patient file to research is Stacy Ardell. Ms. Ardell, a victim of spousal abuse, was seen at the clinic as a walk-in emergency patient. She received a physical examination and an evaluation of her cuts and bruises. An X-ray was performed on her shoulder, revealing a dislocation of the humerus and scapula. Ms. Ardell was transferred to the hospital for treatment. She has insurance coverage through her husband's Tricare policy.

Respond to the following questions and perform the listed skills. *Skills will be accomplished by pairing with a classmate. Role-play the case study where indicated.*

1. Rain Story

   a. Medicaid denied the claim due to improper sequence of billing. After reviewing Rain's patient file, you realize that she has BC/BS as her primary insurance and that Medicaid was billed first. Prepare a new claim form for submittal to BC/BS. Diagnoses: Supervision of high-risk pregnancy with history of abortion, hypothyroidism. Your instructor will provide you with the correct fees.

b. In writing, explain the sequence of billing steps involved when submitting a claim form to a third-party biller and Medicaid.

_____

_____

_____

_____

c. Submit the completed claim form to BC/BS to Dr. Carlson (your instructor) for her signature.

2. Stacy Ardell

a. Access the form titled *Stacy Ardell* from the Forms CD. Using the originally submitted insurance claim form, identify the coding errors.

b. Complete the new claim form with the corrected codes. Submit it to Dr. Carlson for her signature.

c. Respond to the following in writing: What is the relationship between procedure and diagnostic codes?

_____

_____

_____

_____

d. Tricare has also asked for you to submit a more in-depth description of Stacy's injuries. Ask Dr. Carlson (your instructor) so that you can draft a more complete description. Type the draft for Dr. Carlson's signature. This will accompany the new form to be sent to Tricare.

e. After receiving both the updated description and corrected claim form with Dr. Carlson's signature, prepare the documents to be mailed to Tricare.

CASE STUDY 17

Photocopier Maintenance and Repairs

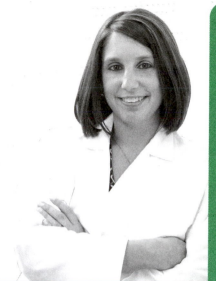

ADMINISTRATIVE

KMC purchased a photocopier machine less than six months ago. The machine is not working properly and continues to feed the paper inappropriately. Mary Colleen Callaghan would like for you to research the contents of the photocopier instruction manual to evaluate any troubleshooting methods.

You have read the manual and attempted to remedy the photocopier machine with several troubleshooting methods to no avail. You inform Mary Colleen that you have tried all troubleshooting methods and that you are fairly sure that repairs will be covered under the product warranty because the machine is less than six months old. She instructs you to call and set up an appointment for repair services.

Respond to the following questions and perform the listed skills. *Skills will be accomplished by pairing with a classmate. Role-play the case study where indicated.*

1. Obtain a copy of KMC's photocopier manual (your instructor will provide this to you).

2. Locate the section that provides information regarding troubleshooting paper jams. In writing, provide Mary Colleen (your instructor) with a brief synopsis of things that may cause the paper to jam.

3. Obtain a copy of the clinic's warranty (your instructor will provide this to you). Determine whether the warranty covers the needed repairs.

4. Locate the name, telephone number, and address of a local repair service that can repair your particular model of photocopier and provide this information to Mary Colleen.

5. Role-play calling to set up an appointment for repair services. Also, establish a routine maintenance schedule for the photocopier.

CASE STUDY **18**

Office Equipment and Computer Concepts

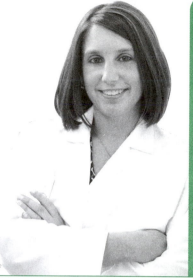

Jason Harper is a new extern who has been assigned to KMC. He will begin his externship in the administrative aspect of the clinic. Mary Colleen Callaghan has requested that you supervise Jason as he becomes familiar with the equipment in the office. She would also like for you to train him on the various computer applications that are used within the clinic.

Respond to the following questions and perform the listed skills. *Skills will be accomplished by pairing with a classmate. Role-play the case study where indicated.*

1. Role-play training Jason on all of the office equipment. Review in detail and demonstrate the usage of the following:

   a. Equipment: computer, calculator, scanners, copy machine, fax machine, and printer

   b. Computer components

   c. Computer applications: database (fields, menu, records, files), networks, security (password), medical practice management software (patient data, report generation)

2. Mary Colleen would like for you to write an informative synopsis of your experience working with and training Jason. She will use it when completing Jason's externship evaluation. Submit the synopsis to Mary Colleen (your instructor).

Name _____ Date _____

CASE STUDY **19**

Scheduling Methods

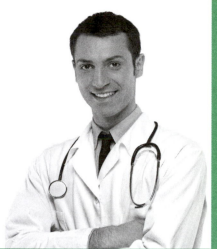

Dr. Greggs has been concerned about the patient wait time and the shortened lunch hours at KMC. Although each health care provider has his or her own scheduling preferences, he has noticed that the current methods are not working. Dr. Greggs would like for you to research the different scheduling methods and determine which would be most beneficial to the clinic. He would like for you to compile the information into a short PowerPoint presentation to be held at the next staff meeting.

Respond to the following questions and perform the listed skills. *Skills will be accomplished by pairing with a classmate. Role-play the case study where indicated.*

1. Research each type of scheduling method.

2. Write a brief description of each scheduling method and submit it to Dr. Greggs (your instructor).

3. Determine the method that you think should be implemented within the clinic based on the number of practitioners and patient volume. State the reason for your choice, in writing, and submit it to Dr. Greggs.

4. Create a short PowerPoint presentation that acts as a descriptor for the various scheduling methods. Conclude with your choice of a scheduling method and provide the reasoning that establishes your choice as the most effective method to implement within the clinic. Present your PowerPoint presentation at the staff meeting (to your classmates and instructor).

CASE STUDY **20**

Managing an Angry Caller

You are answering the telephones this morning at the clinic when a patient calls and begins to accuse the clinic of stealing her money. Hannah Brooks informs you that she made a payment that has not been subtracted from her amount due. You inform her that there have been no payments made to her account for 160 days. She begins raising her voice and states, "I am aware that you assume I haven't made any payments because I received your collection letter last week that my account was past due for 150 days!" Ms. Brooks begins to accuse you of not posting her payment and is relentless in her effort to convince you that she made a payment last month.

You have spoken with Ms. Brooks before about her past-due account and are aware that she recently lost her job and is a single parent. You are also convinced that her angry tone and accusations are the result of frustration from her financial difficulties. You try to explain to Ms. Brooks that you did not receive a payment because you would have credited it to her account immediately. She in return becomes even more defensive and volatile. She threatens to come to the office and cause you bodily harm if you do not fix the situation.

Respond to the following questions and perform the listed skills. *Skills will be accomplished by pairing with a classmate. Role-play the case study where indicated.*

1. Role-play the method for answering and screening five multiple-line telephone calls. Be sure to handle the callers appropriately, such as taking messages, placing callers on hold, or transferring calls to other staff members.

2. Role-play answering the phone and conversing with Hannah. Remember to communicate in a professional manner.

3. Respond to the following questions with detailed answers and submit them to Mary Colleen (your instructor).

   • In what ways is it difficult to maintain professional communication with an angry caller?

   • How can professional communication be adapted to meet the needs of an angry caller?

- What are some things that should be avoided when handling an angry caller?

- How might one proceed with this type of call?

- Should the call be transferred to someone in a higher position?

- If the patient cannot be calmed, what should you do?

- If you feel that Hannah is serious about coming to the clinic and causing you bodily harm, what would your next step be?

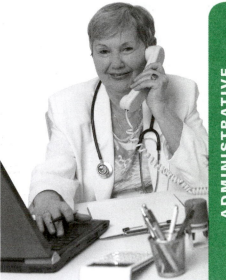

© StockLite/www.Shutterstock.com

CASE STUDY **21**

HIPAA–Privacy and Breach of Confidentiality

Elisa Fox is a well-known reporter and is a patient at KMC. The results from the tests performed during her vaginal examination last week have just been faxed over and the office staff is already speculating on who might have given her gonorrhea. The staff is relentless in pursuit of an answer and has been questioning each other all day. You are concerned that other patients may hear what the diagnosis is and begin to spread this information.

You question the office staff to find out who originally pulled the results off the fax machine and find out that Marcy, your student extern, retrieved the information and started the gossip. She is supposed to be working under your direct supervision and has created a potentially difficult situation for the clinic.

Respond to the following questions and perform the listed skills. *Skills will be accomplished by pairing with a classmate. Role-play the case study where indicated.*

1. Which one of the following would be the most appropriate action in this situation? Defend your response in writing and submit it to Dr. Carlson (your instructor).

   a. Nothing, it will eventually just go away.

   b. Discuss the situation with Marcy.

   c. Call the externship coordinator at Marcy's school and discuss the situation with him or her before speaking with Marcy.

   d. Immediately dismiss Marcy from KMC and post a failing grade on Marcy's externship paperwork. Fax the grade sheet to the school.

2. How do privacy and confidentiality policies promote competent patient care? Does this situation violate any HIPAA policies? If so, which ones? (Respond in writing and submit your answers to your instructor.)

3. What is the proper way to handle a fax? How should this correspondence been received, organized, prioritized, and documented? (Address each question individually in writing and submit your answers to your instructor.)

43

4. Is there a possibility that Marcy will not be allowed to graduate from her medical assistant program because of this indiscretion? Could Marcy lose the ability to certify as a medical assistant? If Marcy has already been certified, is there a possibility she could lose her certification? What are the implications should any of the above occur? (Address each question individually in writing and submit your answers to your instructor.)

5. In the role of the clinic's medical assistant and Marcy's supervisor, role-play a discussion with Marcy regarding this matter. Incorporate the following key elements in the discussion:

   - Display a professional attitude, using professional communication techniques.

   - Discuss accepting responsibility for one's own actions.

   - Discuss the need for staff to support the professional organization and speak with Marcy about how her actions may have impacted her ability and the staff's ability to do so.

   - Discuss how the decisions made by Marcy did or did not promote competent patient care.

   - Discuss how Marcy could have handled the situation using tact, diplomacy, and integrity.

6. In a letter addressed to Dr. Carlson, document the key points of your discussion with Marcy. Send the letter as an e-mail attachment to Dr. Carlson (your instructor).

CASE STUDY **22**

Research and Memo for CLIA and Point-of-Care Testing

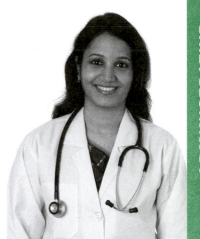

ADMINISTRATIVE

Susah Patel is requesting that you do research regarding updated CLIA guidelines for point-of-care testing. She would like for you to compile a list of point-of-care tests that have been approved for the Physician Office Laboratory (POL) within KMC, and draft any updates to the testing procedures into a memo. Susah is particularly interested in any newly approved CLIA-waived tests. She would like for you to submit your rough draft to her for verification and proofreading.

Susah has verified the information within your memo and has made some notations that she would like you to correct. She also requests that after you have made the changes you submit the information via e-mail to Drs. Carlson, Greggs, Wertz, and Bledsole.

Respond to the following questions and perform the listed skills.

1. Research as needed, compile a list, and draft the memo. Submit it to Susah (your instructor) electronically. Proofread your material carefully.

2. Susah will proofread your first draft and return it to you for corrections.

3. Make corrections and create a final draft to be sent to Drs. Carlson, Greggs, Wertz, Bledsole and Susah (your instructor).

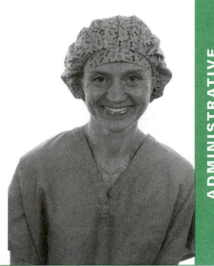

ADMINISTRATIVE

CASE STUDY **23**

Pre-Op Consultation

© rj lerich/www.Shutterstock.com

Wanda Malone is a 67-year-old patient who has come to KMC today for follow-up results to a biopsy performed on a mass located in her left breast. You escort Mrs. Malone to Dr. Wertz's office. Dr. Wertz informs Mrs. Malone that the mass is malignant and that due to the advanced stage of cancer she will need to be scheduled for a lumpectomy next week. Dr. Wertz explains the procedure to Mrs. Malone and informs her that you will be scheduling her surgery with Dr. Robinson, who is a surgeon Dr. Wertz trusts and often refers patients. Dr. Wertz will also be referring Mrs. Malone to an oncologist, Nadine Bradshaw.

You schedule the lumpectomy with Dr. Robinson for next week at the surgical center. Because Dr. Wertz will be assisting, Dr. Robinson's office would like for you to obtain precertification from Medicare for the procedure, perform a pre-op consultation, complete a referral form, and obtain a copy of Mrs. Malone's insurance information. They would like for you to fax the documentation to them by the end of the day in order to establish Mrs. Malone as a patient before her surgery.

Respond to the following questions and perform the listed skills. *Skills will be accomplished by pairing with a classmate. Role-play the case study where indicated.*

1. Obtain Mrs. Malone's chart.

2. Introduce yourself to the patient.

3. Escort Mrs. Malone to Dr. Wertz's office.

4. Role-play the scheduling of the lumpectomy and provide an appointment card and procedure-specific instructions to Mrs. Malone.

5. Role-play preauthorization and precertification from Medicare. (Research the procedure as needed.)

6. Role-play performing a pre-op consultation. (Research the components of a pre-op consultation as needed. Be sure to include questions about advance directives and anatomical gifts.) Remember that Mrs. Malone may be distraught, withdrawn, agitated, and uncooperative or sullen and angry because she has just been diagnosed with cancer.

7. Obtain a copy of Mrs. Malone's insurance card.

8. Obtain the appropriate consent forms. Dr. Wertz will personally explain the surgical consent, but you will need to provide the form to Dr. Wertz.

9. Fax the required information to Dr. Robinson's office.

10. Role-play calling Dr. Bradshaw's office to notify them of Dr. Wertz's referral. Unfortunately, Dr. Bradshaw does not have an available appointment for three months. What would be your next step?

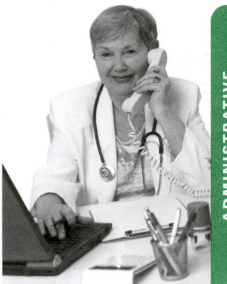

CASE STUDY **24**

Breach of Confidentiality– Intentional Tort

ADMINISTRATIVE

You telephoned Elisa Fox to set up an appointment for which she will be informed of the results of the tests that were performed during her vaginal examination last week. She informs you that her personal information was leaked from your office and that there are other reporters calling her to confirm the information. She informs you that from this point forward she will not maintain contact with KMC unless it is through her lawyers.

You notify Dr. Carlson about the situation and explain that Marcy retrieved the results from the fax machine and began to speculate with other office staff about who could have given Elisa gonorrhea.

Dr. Carlson is reasonably upset and concerned about an upcoming lawsuit for failing to maintain confidentiality. She instructs you to research all plausible repercussions for this breach and to present the information at an emergency staff meeting this afternoon.

Respond to the following questions and perform the listed skills.

1. Research the following and craft a 10–12 slide PowerPoint presentation addressing the following topics and their impact on the current situation:

   - Medical practice acts

   - Physician-patient relationship

   - Responsibility and rights of a patient, physician, and medical assistant

   - Professional liability

   - Maintaining confidentiality

   - Intentional tort: invasion of privacy, slander, and libel

   - Ethics

2. Submit your presentation to Dr. Carlson for review and comment. Be prepared to make a presentation at an emergency staff meeting.

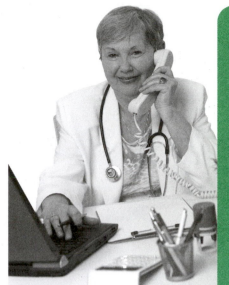

CASE STUDY **25**

Termination of Employment

ADMINISTRATIVE

Barbara has been KMC's administrative medical assistant for the past nine months. She is friendly and outgoing and spends a lot of time talking to the patients before and after the patients' appointments. The patients really enjoy talking to Barbara; even the grumpiest patients seem a little happier. Barbara is a good listener and is very compassionate. She remembers the details of a patient's life that makes each one feel important. She can often be found discussing everything from the latest college football scores to the dance recital of Mrs. Olsen's granddaughter.

This morning, as Dr. Carlson was walking by the front desk, she overheard Barbara telling George Heinzelmen, a patient, how sad she was to have heard that another patient at the clinic, Angie Johnson, had just been diagnosed as HIV positive. Dr. Carlson has not given Angie the test results yet.

After Mr. Heinzelmen went to sit in the waiting area, Dr. Carlson harshly asks Barbara to come to her office. Dr. Carlson informs Barbara that she overheard the conversation discussing one patient's test results with another patient. Dr. Carlson reminds Barbara that she has violated several legal and ethical regulations, not to mention the clinic's employment policies and procedures. Dr. Carlson then terminates Barbara's employment at KMC, effective immediately.

Respond to the following questions and perform the listed skills. *Skills will be accomplished by pairing with a classmate. Role-play the case study where indicated.*

1. Role-play with your instructor, or a classmate (if directed), the discussion between Dr. Carlson and Barbara. Your role is to play Barbara, defending your actions.

2. On what grounds has Barbara's employment been terminated?

   _____

   _____

   _____

   _____

3. Can Dr. Carlson legally terminate Barbara's employment? Why or why not? (Research, as necessary, the employment laws governing this situation in your state.)

_____

_____

_____

_____

4. Is Dr. Carlson legally or ethically bound to tell Angie that this incidence occurred? Why or why not?

_____

_____

_____

_____

5. Is Dr. Carlson allowed to provide Angie with a diagnosis over the telephone due to the circumstances? (If so, role-play step 8 using the telephone; if not, role-play the situation in person.)

_____

_____

_____

_____

6. Must Angie's diagnosis be reported to any outside agency(s)? If so, which agency(s)?

_____

_____

_____

_____

7. Has Angie's criminal and/or civil rights been violated? (Research as necessary.) Provide one real-life criminal and/or civil court case substantiating your response. Provide the names of the plaintiff and the defendant, a case number, the name of the judge who tried the case, the state where the case was tried, and the outcome.

_____

_____

_____

_____

8. Role-play with a classmate the discussion between Dr. Carlson and Angie. Include a discussion on the HIV-positive diagnosis, assuming that Dr. Carlson is obligated to inform Angie of the breach of confidentiality.

9. Observe another pair of classmates role-playing step 8 and write a one-paragraph synopsis evaluating the verbal and nonverbal communication that occurred. Submit your synopsis to your instructor.

_____

_____

_____

_____

10. Create an entry for KMC's employment policy and procedure manual, outlining the grounds for termination based on the legal grounds for termination in your state. Specifically address "Breach of Confidentiality." Submit it to your instructor.

CASE STUDY 26

Informational Report–FDA Guidelines

Marcy has been questioning you about the involvement of the FDA within the clinical environment. You respond by asking her to research the role that the FDA plays within the clinic and any FDA guidelines that are pertinent to the functioning of the clinic. You request that she hand deliver her information to you in the form of a report.

Marcy has followed through with your request and has submitted an informative report about her findings. You found her report to be accurate and would like for her to present the information to the employees during a staff meeting this afternoon.

Respond to the following questions and perform the listed skills. *Skills will be accomplished by pairing with a classmate. Role-play the case study where indicated.*

1. Role-play the conversation between you and Marcy.

2. Research what role the FDA plays in a physician's clinic. Include in your research any FDA guidelines that are pertinent to the functioning of the clinic.

3. Write a two-page report on your findings. Submit your report to a classmate who will assume the role of your supervisor. You will also be required to assume the role of another classmate's supervisor. In the role of the supervisor, review Marcy's report. Use appropriate proofreading symbols and make constructive comments regarding overall content and presentation. Submit the first draft of the report with your proofreading marks and comments to Susah (your instructor).

4. Make a brief (two-minute) presentation to a small group of classmates or the entire class, based on direction from your instructor.

CASE STUDY **27**

Medical Liability Coverage

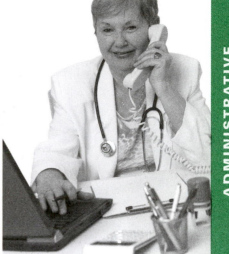

ADMINISTRATIVE

Elisa Fox has informed KMC that she will be contacting a lawyer for the invasion of privacy and breach of confidentiality that took place within the clinic. Dr. Carlson has asked you to verify the amount of liability coverage that the clinic currently maintains. (Ask your instructor for this amount.) The policy has been renewed but there may be other types of coverage that are available for any future issues. Dr. Carlson would also like you to locate current information and rates on the types of coverage that are available and requests that you compile your information into a professional spreadsheet and then to transfer it to her personal flash drive. She will present the information to the other physicians tomorrow morning.

Respond to the following questions and perform the listed skills.

1. Research and compile the following information into a spreadsheet:

   • Current information on medical liability coverage

   • Information for at least three types of coverage

   • Rates for at least three types of coverage

2. Compare and contrast the types of medical liability coverage and create a graph within the spreadsheet that corresponds with this information.

3. Save the spreadsheet onto a flash drive and submit the flash drive to Dr. Carlson (your instructor).

CASE STUDY **28**

ADA–Wheelchair Accessibility

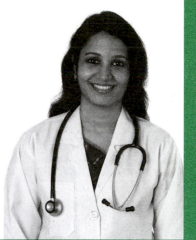

ADMINISTRATIVE

Susah Patel is requesting that you do research regarding updated ADA guidelines for doorway entryways, hallways, and wheelchair access. She wants to ensure that the clinic is up to date on the current requirements. Susah would like for you to submit your research via electronic mail.

Respond to the following questions and perform the listed skills.

1. Research and collect data from a minimum of two resources. Prepare a written report to give to Susah (your instructor). Cite your resources. Send the report electronically as an attachment.

2. After reviewing the report, Susah has asked you to physically measure a minimum of three doorways and two hallways to ensure that they meet the ADA standards. She would also like for you to provide her with a hand-drawn map of the clinic's (your school's) wheelchair access.

3. You discover that two of the three doorways are inadequate for wheelchair access. What would need to be done to make improvements to meet the requirements? Each doorway is 2.6 inches too narrow.

4. Susah would like for you to research the cost involved in making the improvements.

5. What might be some alternatives you can suggest to Susah to accommodate wheelchair access without widening the doors?

6. If you do not make the improvements, what might the repercussions be?

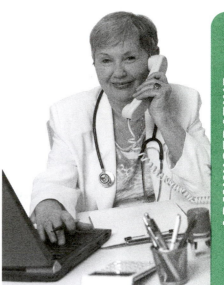

CASE STUDY **29**

Patient Education, Community Support Groups, Stages of Grief

ADMINISTRATIVE

Dr. Carlson has just informed Angie Johnson that she is HIV positive. She has also told Angie about the breach of confidentiality incident. Instead of being furious, Angie remains very quiet and in control. Dr. Carlson asks you to join her and Angie in her office. Angie says she understands that her HIV-positive status could develop into AIDS and that there is no cure. Angie shares with you and Dr. Carlson that she only has had sexual intercourse with her husband; she has never used drugs and is not occupationally exposed to blood or other body fluids. Angie does not know how she could have contracted HIV. She has two small children, ages 5 and 2. Angie begins to cry. Dr. Carlson asks you to comfort Angie and listen to her concerns. She would like for you to explain to Angie the steps in the grief process and to answer any of her questions regarding this. Dr. Carlson also asks that you provide Angie with information about support groups in the community. Dr. Carlson would like to see Angie back at KMC in two weeks.

Respond to the following questions and perform the listed skills. *Skills will be accomplished by pairing with a classmate. Role-play the case study where indicated.*

1. Role-play the discussion with Angie. Note Angie's verbal and nonverbal communication. (Note: Do not begin the role-play activity until you have the information required for steps 1b–d available.)

   a. Comfort Angie and listen to her concerns, responding appropriately.

   b. Explain the steps in the grief process and answer any questions. (Research as necessary.)

   c. Explain to Angie what HIV is; include signs and symptoms, how the disease progresses, what body systems are involved, and the current treatment and prognosis. Angie is very confused on how she could have contracted HIV. Discuss with Angie the possible sources of transmission. (Research as necessary.)

   d. Provide Angie with information on support groups in your community. (Research as necessary.)

2. What defense mechanism is Angie displaying? What is the best way to work with a patient using this defense mechanism?

_____

_____

_____

_____

3. Angie is an existing patient. Document any of Angie's concerns and comments (verbal communication) and her demeanor (nonverbal communication) on a Progress Note form.

CASE STUDY **30**

Policy and Procedure Manual and Notification Letter

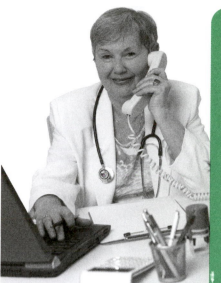

ADMINISTRATIVE

Dr. Carlson is thankful for all of the research and effort you have put into the pending lawsuit by Elisa Fox concerning invasion of privacy and a breach of confidentiality. However, she is asking that you follow through with two more requests to wrap up your research. She would like for you to develop a formal document to be inserted into the KMC policy and procedure manual. She would like for you to submit your rough draft to her for proofreading and approval.

After approval of your document and the correction of any notations, Dr. Carlson would like for you to create a formal letter to be signed by all the physicians and distributed to every member of the staff. The letter will serve as a notice about the addition to the policy and procedure manual and will inform the staff about any disciplinary actions that will occur if the policy is violated.

Your instructor will assign you to a team to work on this case study. Respond to the following questions and perform the listed skills. *Skills will be accomplished by pairing with a classmate. Role-play the case study where indicated.*

1. Gather all information you have collected (as a team) relating to the Elisa Fox case studies. Create a policy and procedure manual formal document using the collective data of all members of the team.

2. Submit the first draft of the document via e-mail to Dr. Carlson (your instructor will supply you with an address). Use the watermark function to notate that this is the first draft of the document. Dr. Carlson will proofread your document and make suggestions for improvements.

3. When the first draft of your document is returned make the required corrections and submit your final draft.

4. Write a formal letter addressed to the entire staff of the clinic to serve as notice of the addition to the policy and procedure manual. Briefly describe the key points of the new document. Include the disciplinary actions.

5. Three employees are on vacation or leave. Dr. Carlson feels that it is important enough to mail a copy of the letter to each employee at his or her home address, using the U.S. Postal Service. Prepare a copy of the letter to be mailed to the following employees: Sarah Mickelson, Addie Cabot, and Marc Elias. Obtain their addresses from employee records (create on your own).

6. Use a postal machine or meter to ready the mail for delivery.

CASE STUDY 31

OSHA–Biohazardous Waste Research and Report

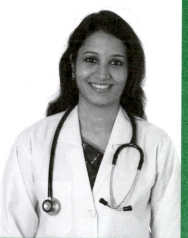

© SnowWhiteImages/www.Shutterstock.com

Susah Patel is requesting that you do research regarding updated OSHA guidelines for the disposal of biohazardous waste. She wants to ensure that KMC is up to date on the current requirements. Susah would like for you to submit your research to her in the form of a report. She would also like you to include your thoughts on how these changes should be made. Submit your report as an attachment to an e-mail.

Respond to the following questions and perform the listed skills.

1. Research OSHA guidelines and requirements for any updates regarding the disposal of biohazardous waste. Your research should include any updates within the last six months.

2. Compile your research into a 1,000-word report using MLA or APA format (which your instructor will determine) and submit it to Susah (your instructor) for evaluation. Your report will be graded on content, correct use of medical terminology, sentence structure, grammar, and punctuation. Be sure to cite your references and proofread your report for errors before submittal.

3. Include at least three ideas that indicate your thoughts on implementing the required OSHA updates to the clinic. These ideas should be placed at the end of your report.

ADMINISTRATIVE

CASE STUDY **32**

OSHA–Office Memo

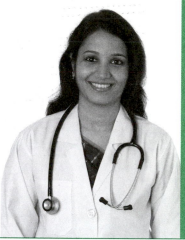

ADMINISTRATIVE

Susah has read your OSHA report (refer to Case Study 31) and has spoken with the physicians about the changes that need to be made regarding the updates for the disposal of biohazardous material. They were impressed with your ideas and would like for you to create and distribute an office memo indicating the new guidelines and the course of action for implementing the changes. Susah has returned your report with some changes that need to be made (your instructor will mark these). She would like for you to be aware of the changes when you are creating your memo.

Respond to the following questions and perform the listed skills.

1. Using your previous researched information and your report from Case Study 31 as a reference, create a 300-word office memo (using MLA or APA format) that indicates the updates required by OSHA and how the clinic is going to implement the changes necessary. Your memo will be graded on content, correct use of medical terminology, sentence structure, grammar, and punctuation. Be sure to cite your references and proofread your memo for errors before distribution (to your instructor).

2. Submit your written response (on a separate paper) to the following questions with your memo.

   a. What are the various methods for distributing a memo throughout the clinic?

   b. In your opinion, which method of delivery is the most effective? Why?

   c. Are there any risks associated with memo delivery methods?

   d. What type of information should not be included in an intraoffice memo?

   e. How are intraoffice communications effective?

67

CASE STUDY **33**

Wellness Physical Examination, Patient Assessment

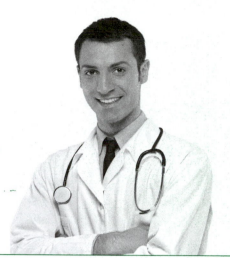

© Ljupco Smokovski/www.Shutterstock.com

Abigail Johansson, a 16-year-old female, has just moved to town. Her mother called KMC and scheduled an appointment for Abigail for a wellness physical, a requirement before enrolling in her new school. Abigail's appointment is today. Before Dr. Greggs's examination, you are required to obtain a medical history and perform a patient assessment, which includes height; weight; temperature, pulse, respiration (TPR); and blood pressure.

Respond to the following questions and perform the listed skills as ordered by Dr. Greggs. All charts and SOAP Note forms will be submitted to Dr. Greggs (your instructor) for review and evaluation. *Skills will be accomplished by pairing with a classmate. Role-play the case study where indicated.*

1. Establish a new-patient chart. (This chart will be created for yourself as if you were the new patient. Note: All procedures and results will be documented in this "patient" chart.)

   a. Include the following items: folder, label with the name properly indexed, date label, allergy label as appropriate, Patient Information form, Medical History form, Consent for Treatment form, Medication Administration form, Privacy Act form, Authorization for Disclosure of Information form, Patient Authorization form, Laboratory Report form (shingled), and a SOAP Note form.

   b. Complete all forms by interviewing a classmate.

   c. You may use your personal information or you can create fictitious information.

   d. Your instructor may also (or alternatively) elect to have you input the patient information into electronic health records (EHR) software. Record all procedures and results on a SOAP Note form and/or input the information into EHR software in the patient's electronic chart.

2. Perform medical aseptic hand hygiene and use standard precautions as appropriate.

3. Assemble equipment and supplies.

4. Introduce yourself to the patient.

5. Obtain the proper intake information.

6. Explain the procedure(s).

7. Perform patient assessment, including height, weight, TPR, and blood pressure. Use an oral thermometer to obtain the patient's temperature.

8. Provide the patient with instructions for proper positioning and draping in preparation for the wellness physical examination.

9. Properly position and drape the patient for the physical examination.

10. Perform proper hand hygiene. Properly dispose of all waste materials.

11. Record all procedures and results on a SOAP Note form and/or in the patient's electronic chart. Submit all documentation to Dr. Greggs (your instructor) for review and evaluation.

12. What supplies and equipment should you have available for Dr. Greggs to complete the physical examination?

_____

_____

_____

_____

CASE STUDY **34**

Patient Education, Patient Assessment

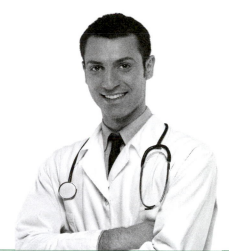

© Ljupco Smokovski/www.Shutterstock.com

CLINICAL

James Fowler, a regular patient of Dr. Greggs, is an African American male in his mid-50s. He has smoked two packs of cigarettes a day for just over 25 years. He has recently developed a chronic cough and is concerned enough that he may quit smoking. James is also significantly overweight; he is 5′8″ tall and at his last office visit he weighed 265 lb. While his blood pressure has been stable for the last few years, Dr. Greggs would like for James to lose some weight as well as quit smoking. Changing his eating habits and quitting smoking at the same time is more than James believes he can accomplish. Dr. Greggs has requested that you measure James's vital signs as well as his height and weight.

Today when you measured James's vital signs his blood pressure has jumped from 140/90 to 156/100, his weight has increased five pounds, and his heart rate is slightly increased. You believe that with Dr. Greggs's permission, you may be able to provide advice to James to help him change his lifestyle.

Respond to the following questions and perform the listed skills as ordered by Dr. Greggs. *Skills will be accomplished by pairing with a classmate. Role-play the case study where indicated.*

1. Perform medical aseptic hand hygiene and use standard precautions as appropriate.

2. Assemble equipment and supplies.

3. Introduce yourself to the patient.

4. Obtain the proper intake information.

5. Explain the procedure(s).

6. Perform patient assessment, including height, weight, TPR, and blood pressure. Use a tympanic thermometer to obtain the patient's temperature. Use a large blood pressure cuff.

7. Perform proper hand hygiene. Properly dispose of all waste materials.

8. Is a blood pressure reading of 156/100 a cause for concern? Should you take a second reading to confirm the results?

_____

_____

_____

_____

9. When measuring blood pressure, what role does the size of the blood pressure cuff play? Should you have used a regular-size blood pressure cuff to measure James's blood pressure? Explain your answer.

_____

_____

_____

_____

10. Role-play the education that you would give James regarding his required lifestyle changes. Specifically address hypertension, weight loss, and smoking cessation. (Research options for weight loss and quitting smoking.)

11. Review your knowledge of hypertension and role-play a discussion regarding the four types of hypertension and their specific characteristics with Dr. Greggs.

12. Record all procedures and results on a SOAP Note form and/or input the information into the patient's electronic chart. Submit all documentation to Dr. Greggs (your instructor) for review and evaluation.

CASE STUDY **35**

Capillary Puncture, Pediatric Patient

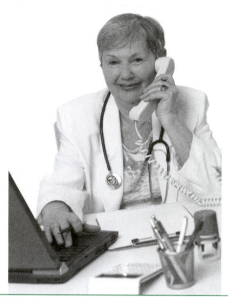

© StockLite/www.Shutterstock.com

CLINICAL

Chrissie Henkle, a 9-year-old young girl with a mental challenge, has an appointment today. Chrissie is an established patient. Dr. Carlson has requested a stat Hct, Hgb, and blood glucose. Chrissie is sitting on her mother's lap in the draw chair. As you start to assemble your equipment and supplies, she becomes agitated. She tries to negotiate with her mom about coming back later. Chrissie's mom tells her that she has to have the test done now so the physician can make her feel better. You try to establish a rapport with Chrissie, telling her that it is not going to hurt and that if she is good you will give her stickers when she is done. You convince her to let you perform a finger stick. You know that you probably are only going to have one chance. You have assembled all of the equipment, washed your hands, donned gloves, and are starting to cleanse the finger when Chrissie becomes more and more agitated, arching her back and pulling away from you.

Respond to the following questions and perform the listed skills as ordered by Dr. Carlson. *Skills will be accomplished by pairing with a classmate. Role-play the case study where indicated.*

1. Perform medical aseptic hand hygiene and use standard precautions as appropriate.

2. Assemble equipment and supplies.

3. Introduce yourself to the patient.

4. Obtain the proper intake information.

5. Role-play with a classmate establishing a rapport with Chrissie.

6. Explain the procedure(s).

7. Perform patient assessment including height, weight, TPR, and blood pressure. Use a tympanic thermometer to obtain the patient's temperature.

8. Because this collection has been ordered stat, what should you do?

_____

_____

_____

_____

9. What error did you initially make with Chrissie?

_____

_____

_____

_____

10. Perform a capillary puncture. Fill two microhematocrit tubes. (You will not actually be performing the laboratory tests on this patient.)

11. Perform proper hand hygiene. Properly dispose of all waste materials.

12. Document all procedures and results. Record all procedures and results on a SOAP Note form and/or the patient's electronic chart. Submit all documentation to Dr. Carlson (your instructor) for review and evaluation.

13. Role-play this case study with a different classmate playing the role of a "non-agitated Chrissie." Document "nonagitated Chrissie's" procedures and results on the same SOAP Note form, identifying the results as Chrissie #2.

CASE STUDY **36**

Hypertension–Patient Assessment (Part 1)

CLINICAL

Sylvia Newman, a 52-year-old female patient, comes into the clinic every Monday, Wednesday, and Friday at 12:30 p.m. for a blood pressure check. Her blood pressure has been intermittently high over the past six months. Dr. Wertz prescribed her blood pressure medication two weeks ago and it seems to be keeping her blood pressure within normal limits. However, today she seems rather upset and in a hurry. She tells you that she needs to be seen immediately, because she needs to get back to work as soon as possible. As you are taking her back to the examination room, she tells you that the blood pressure medication the doctor prescribed for her is making her nauseous and that she has not taken her pills for the past two days.

Respond to the following questions and perform the listed skills. *Skills will be accomplished by pairing with a classmate. Role-play the case study where indicated.*

1. Perform medical aseptic hand hygiene and use standard precautions as appropriate.

2. Assemble equipment and supplies.

3. Introduce yourself to the patient.

4. Obtain the proper intake information.

5. Explain the procedure(s).

6. Perform patient assessment including height, weight, TPR, and blood pressure. Use an oral thermometer to obtain the patient's temperature.

7. Perform proper hand hygiene. Properly dispose of all waste materials.

8. Provide appropriate patient instructions.

9. Sylvia's blood pressure has been averaging 134/86. What result should you expect to see today?

_____

_____

_____

_____

10. Record the actual vital sign results obtained on a classmate. Then record the following results in parentheses as Sylvia's results.

   a. Temperature: normal body temperature

   b. Pulse: 24 beats for 15 seconds

   c. Respiration: 22

   d. Blood Pressure: 194/102

11. What should your next course of action be? If Sylvia is unwilling to comply with this course of action, what would you do next? (Research as needed.)

_____

_____

_____

_____

12. Dialogue step 10 verbally with a classmate, and then document the conversation in Sylvia's chart.

13. Record all procedures and results on a SOAP Note form and/or the patient's electronic chart. Submit all documentation to Dr. Wertz (your instructor) for review and evaluation.

CASE STUDY **37**

Principles of Infection Control

You are still responsible for supervising and training Jason on the various duties of medical assisting. You explain to Jason that KMC inventories instruments on a monthly basis to verify that the sterilization and disinfection dates are current. Upon inspection, you find two surgical instrument packs (a cervical tenaculum and a curette) that need to be sterilized again.

Respond to the following questions and perform the listed skills. *Skills will be accomplished by pairing with a classmate. Role-play the case study where indicated.*

1. Role-play with Jason the office policy of completing inventories of instruments and instrument packs. Explain how long an instrument pack may be stored before it is not considered sterile. Describe the process that is required for the instruments to be sterilized again.

2. Perform an inventory of the clinic's (your classroom's) instruments and instrument packs.

3. Perform medical aseptic hand hygiene and use standard precautions as appropriate.

4. Unwrap surgical packs and discard any disposable items.

5. Sanitize and disinfect the instruments.

6. Prepare new packs for sterilization.

7. Sterilize instrument packs in the autoclave.

8. Submit both surgical packs (Jason's and yours) to Mary Colleen Callaghan (your instructor) for final approval and grading.

CASE STUDY 38

Well-Baby Check, Pediatrics

© StockLite/www.Shutterstock.com

Taylor Hunter is a new patient to the clinic. She is six weeks old and due for her well-baby examination. Dr. Carlson delivered her and Taylor's mom, Kim Hunter, has requested Dr. Carlson continue caring for her.

Respond to the following questions and perform the listed skills as ordered by Dr. Carlson. *Skills will be accomplished by pairing with a classmate. Role-play the case study where indicated.*

1. Taylor Hunter has not been seen at KMC before. Create a new patient chart (your instructor will direct whether it should be a paper or electronic chart). If you were creating a new patient paper chart for Taylor, what forms would you need to complete her file?

   _____

   _____

   _____

   _____

2. Perform medical aseptic hand hygiene and use standard precautions as appropriate.

3. Assemble equipment and supplies.

4. Introduce yourself to the patient and the patient's mother.

5. Obtain the proper intake information.

6. Obtain proper consent(s).

7. Perform patient assessment including length, weight, head circumference, and temperature. Use a tympanic thermometer to obtain the patient's temperature.

8. Ask Mrs. Hunter to disrobe Taylor for the examination. After the examination Mrs. Hunter can redress Taylor.

9. What supplies and equipment should you have available for Dr. Carlson to complete the physical examination?

_____

_____

_____

_____

10. Chart Taylor's length, weight, and head circumference on the appropriate growth chart.

11. Perform proper hand hygiene. Properly dispose of all waste materials.

12. Record all procedures and results on a SOAP Note form and/or the patient's electronic chart.

13. Submit all documentation to Dr. Carlson (your instructor) for review and evaluation.

CASE STUDY **39**

Hypertension–Patient Assessment (Part 2)

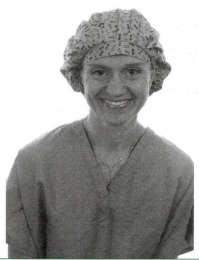

© rj lerich/www.Shutterstock.com

Sylvia Newman, a 52-year-old female patient, comes into KMC every Monday, Wednesday, and Friday at 12:30 p.m. for a blood pressure check. Her blood pressure has been intermittently high over the past six months and Dr. Wertz prescribed her blood pressure medication two weeks ago. In Case Study 36, Sylvia had been upset and in a hurry and had gone off her blood pressure medication. Pull her chart notes from Case Study 36 and document this week's blood pressure readings. This will be accomplished by performing a full patient assessment on three separate classmates (one classmate for Monday, one for Wednesday, and one for Friday). Record the results on Sylvia's SOAP Notes and/or electronic chart on the appropriate days.

Respond to the following questions and perform the listed skills. *Skills will be accomplished by pairing with a classmate. Role-play the case study where indicated.*

1. Perform medical aseptic hand hygiene and use standard precautions as appropriate.

2. Assemble equipment and supplies.

3. Introduce yourself to the patient.

4. Obtain the proper intake information.

5. Explain the procedure(s).

6. Perform three patient assessments (include height, weight, TPR, and blood pressure). Use the tympanic thermometer to obtain the patient's temperature.

7. Provide appropriate patient instructions.

8. Perform proper hand hygiene. Properly dispose of all waste materials.

9. Record the actual vital signs of classmates on Sylvia's SOAP Notes and/or electronic chart.

10. Assess Sylvia's blood pressure results and write a dialogue describing your conversation about Sylvia's results with Dr. Wertz. Verbally discuss your assessment with Dr. Wertz (your instructor).

11. Record all procedures and results on a SOAP Note form and/or the patient's electronic chart. Submit all documentation to Dr. Wertz (your instructor) for review and evaluation.

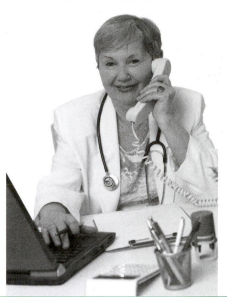

CASE STUDY **40**

Capillary Puncture, INR Point-of-Care Testing

CLINICAL

Donald Williams is a 56-year-old new patient of Dr. Carlson. Dr. Carlson has ordered an international normalized ratio (INR) test. An INR blood test, which checks the blood's ability to clot, can be performed as a Point-of-Care test, either on capillary or venous blood. You ask Mr. Williams his preference, and he responds "finger stick."

Respond to the following questions and perform the listed skills as ordered by Dr. Carlson. *Skills will be accomplished by pairing with a classmate. Role-play the case study where indicated.*

1. Create a new patient chart for Mr. Williams (your instructor will direct whether it should be a paper or an electronic chart). What forms will require Mr. Williams's signature?

   _____

   _____

   _____

   _____

2. Perform medical aseptic hand hygiene and use standard precautions as appropriate.

3. Assemble equipment and supplies.

4. Introduce yourself to the patient.

5. Obtain the proper intake information.

6. Explain the procedure(s).

7. Perform patient assessment including height, weight, TPR, and blood pressure. Use a temporal scanner infrared thermometer to obtain the patient's temperature.

8. Prepare Mr. Williams for his laboratory test.

9. Perform capillary puncture.

10. Perform the INR Point-of-Care test.

11. What is a normal INR in a healthy adult? (Research as necessary.)

_____

_____

_____

_____

12. Perform proper hand hygiene. Properly dispose of all waste materials.

13. Record all procedures and results on a SOAP Note form and/or the patient's electronic chart. Submit all documentation to Dr. Carlson (your instructor) for review and evaluation.

CASE STUDY 41

Pap Smear and Breast Examination

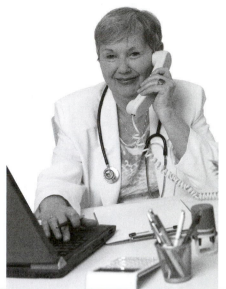

© StockLite/www.Shutterstock.com

Veronica Staples has called KMC with complaints of heavy and very painful menstruation cycles combined with intermittent spotting. You schedule her for an appointment with Dr. Carlson for a pelvic examination, Pap smear, and breast examination. Veronica is 17 years old and a new patient. She has never had a pelvic examination, Pap smear, or breast examination before. You provide Veronica with instructions concerning preparation for her appointment and schedule her appointment for tomorrow.

Ms. Staples arrives 20 minutes early for her appointment and begins filling out the required paperwork. During her patient assessment she confesses that she is quite nervous about her procedures today. She is not sure what to expect and is wondering if you will explain it to her before the doctor comes in.

Respond to the following questions and perform the listed skills as ordered by Dr. Carlson. *Skills will be accomplished by pairing with a classmate. Role-play the case study where indicated.*

1. Role-play with a classmate the scheduling of Veronica's appointment via telephone.

2. What information will you need to obtain from Veronica when making the appointment? Respond in writing and address it during the role-play.

   _____

   _____

   _____

   _____

3. What instructions will you provide to Veronica on the telephone regarding her appointment for her pelvic examination, Pap smear, and breast examination? Respond in writing and address them during the role-play. (Research as necessary.)

_____

_____

_____

_____

4. Use proper telephone etiquette during role-play in steps 1–3.

5. Create a new patient chart (your instructor will direct whether it should be a paper or an electronic chart).

6. Perform medical aseptic hand hygiene and use standard precautions as appropriate.

7. Assemble equipment and supplies. Respond in writing to the following question: What equipment and supplies are needed for these procedures? (Research as necessary.)

_____

_____

_____

_____

8. Escort Veronica to the examination room and introduce yourself.

9. Obtain and document the proper intake information. Verify that the instructions given before the appointment have been followed.

10. Obtain proper consents.

11. Will Veronica require a parent or guardian to be present during the examinations? Research the laws in your state.

_____

_____

_____

_____

12. Perform patient assessment including height, weight, TPR, and blood pressure. Use a tympanic thermometer to obtain the patient's temperature.

13. Ask Veronica to disrobe and provide her with a gown and drape.

14. Explain the procedures to Veronica.

15. For each procedure, identify how Veronica should be positioned and how the gown and drape should be placed. Respond in writing and address them during the role-play.

_____

_____

_____

_____

16. Assist the physician in the procedures as required.

17. Prepare the slide/vial for the Pap smear to be sent to the laboratory.

18. Perform proper hand hygiene. Properly dispose of all waste materials.

19. Inform the patient about what to expect regarding any symptoms she may experience from the procedures and when to expect results.

20. Record all procedures on a SOAP Note form and/or the patient's electronic chart. Submit all documentation to Dr. Carlson (your instructor) for review and evaluation.

CASE STUDY **42**

Preoperative Examination and Laboratory Tests

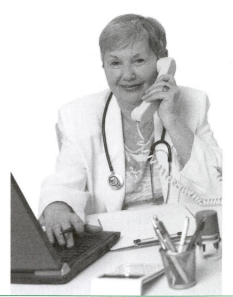

© StockLite/www.shutterstock.com

Warren Black is a 32-year-old male patient of Dr. Carlson's. Dr. Carlson will be performing rotator cuff repair on Mr. Black's shoulder next Thursday morning. Mr. Black is in the clinic today for his preoperative work-up. Because Mr. Black smokes one to two packs of cigarettes per day, Dr. Carlson has requested a complete physical examination, blood work, and a chest X-ray as part of the preoperative procedures.

    Dr. Carlson will do the physical examination; you will be required to do the patient assessment and draw blood for the following tests: CBC, Chem-20 Panel, and bleeding time. The blood will be sent to an independent laboratory for testing. The chest X-ray will need to be scheduled for Mr. Black at the hospital. You will also need to reserve an operating room for the surgery. Mr. Black will require an overnight stay in the hospital. His insurance will not pay for a private room or for more than a one-night stay for this type of surgery. Be sure to obtain the appropriate consents while Mr. Black is at the clinic.

Respond to the following questions and perform the listed skills as ordered by Dr. Carlson. *Skills will be accomplished by pairing with a classmate. Role-play the case study where indicated.*

1. Perform medical aseptic hand hygiene and use standard precautions as appropriate.

2. Assemble equipment and supplies.

3. Introduce yourself to the patient.

4. Obtain the proper intake information.

5. Explain the procedure(s).

6. Obtain the proper consent(s).

7. Perform patient assessment including height, weight, TPR, and blood pressure. Use an oral thermometer to obtain the patient's temperature.

8. Provide appropriate patient instructions.

9. Perform the venipuncture.

10. Draw the correct number and color-topped tubes for each test ordered. (Research as needed.)

11. Perform proper hand hygiene. Properly dispose of all waste materials.

12. What supplies and equipment should be available for Dr. Carlson to complete the physical examination? (Research as needed.)

_____

_____

_____

_____

13. Package specimens to be sent to the laboratory for testing.

14. Schedule chest X-ray, operating room, and overnight stay. What information will be needed to schedule these events? (Research as needed.) Verbally record scheduling the chest X-ray, operating room, and hospital stay for Dr. Carlson's review and evaluation.

_____

_____

_____

_____

15. Why is Dr. Carlson ordering these specific laboratory tests? What are the normal values for this patient? (Research as needed.)

_____

_____

_____

_____

16. Record all procedures and results on a SOAP Note form and/or the patient's electronic chart. Submit all documentation to Dr. Carlson (your instructor) for review and evaluation.

CASE STUDY 43

Vaccinations, Influenza

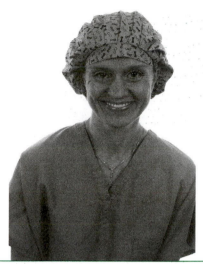

© rj lerich/www.Shutterstock.com

It is flu season again, and KMC is offering influenza vaccines to businesses at very reasonable rates. Today you and your coworkers will be giving vaccinations at the electric company. There are 16 employees signed up to receive vaccinations; you will be giving three of them. Because the employees of the electric company are not patients of KMC, no patient charts will need to be created. However, each vaccination must be documented on an individual SOAP Note form (hardcopy). The form must have the employee's name, date of birth, and a contact telephone number. The name of the vaccination, dose, route, and location of administration as well as the date, time, and your initials must be included on the progress note. Each employee must also sign a consent form. Dr. Wertz has ordered Fluvirin 1 mg to be used as the vaccination. Dr. Wertz requires individuals to remain in the area for five minutes after the vaccination in case of reactions.

Respond to the following questions and perform the listed skills as ordered by Dr. Wertz. *Skills will be accomplished by pairing with a classmate(s). Role-play the case study where indicated.*

1. Perform medical aseptic hand hygiene and use standard precautions as appropriate.

2. Assemble equipment and supplies.

3. Introduce yourself to the employees/patients.

4. Obtain the proper intake information.

5. Explain the procedure(s) to the employees including the risks and side effects of the vaccinations. (Research as needed.)

6. Obtain proper consent from each patient.

7. Perform patient assessments including TPR and blood pressure. Use an oral thermometer to obtain the temperature of the patients.

8. Perform the vaccinations.

9. Perform proper hand hygiene. Properly dispose of all waste materials.

10. Document all procedures and results. Record all procedures and results on a SOAP Note form. Submit all documentation to Dr. Wertz (your instructor) for review and evaluation.

11. Three minutes after receiving the vaccination, the second employee, starts to experience shortness of breath (SOB), mucosal swelling, and hives. What condition is the employee experiencing? (Research answers to question 11 as needed.)

   a. What medications would be administered to combat this condition under a physician's order?

   _____

   _____

   _____

   _____

   b. What route would these medications be given by?

   _____

   _____

   _____

   _____

   c. What steps would you follow upon the patient's reaction to the vaccination?

   _____

   _____

   _____

   _____

   d. What specific information should have been obtained before the vaccination was administered?

   _____

   _____

   _____

   _____

   e. Provide follow-up documentation for this incident on the SOAP Note form for the second employee.

CASE STUDY 44

Digestive Disorder

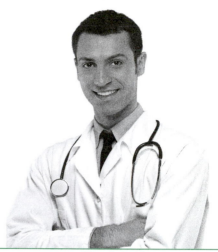

© Ljupco Smokovski/www.Shutterstock.com

Gideon Straus is a 25-year-old male. He has not been seen at the clinic before. Gideon has been experiencing diarrhea, rectal bleeding, and pain in his lower abdomen for quite some time.

Dr. Greggs would like you to obtain a complete family history and any personal data that seem pertinent to today's complaints. You find that Gideon's brother was diagnosed with Crohn's disease last year. You record the information and notify Dr. Greggs of your findings.

Dr. Greggs attends to Gideon. He performs a physical examination and a digital rectal examination. He concludes that some further testing needs to be done. Dr. Greggs has ordered a CBC to check for a raised white blood cell count and to verify that anemia is not present. He would also like you to explain to Gideon how to collect a stool sample for a guaiac test and to provide him with the supplies to do so. Finally, Dr. Greggs would like for you to schedule an appointment for Gideon to have a sigmoidoscopy.

Respond to the following questions and perform the listed skills as ordered by Dr. Greggs. *Skills will be accomplished by pairing with a classmate. Role-play the case study where indicated.*

1. Gideon is a new patient and will require a new chart.

2. Perform medical aseptic hand hygiene and use standard precautions as appropriate.

3. Assemble equipment and supplies.

4. Escort Gideon to the examination room and introduce yourself.

5. Obtain and document the proper intake information.

6. Obtain the proper consent(s).

7. Perform patient assessment including height, weight, TPR, and blood pressure. Use an oral thermometer to obtain the patient's temperature.

8. Provide Gideon with a gown or drape and ask him to disrobe appropriately for the examination being performed.

9. Assist Dr. Greggs in the procedure(s), as needed.

10. Perform the venipuncture, collecting the correct number and color-topped tubes for the requested laboratory tests. Identify the correct order of draw. Send the specimens to the laboratory for processing. (Note: Your instructor will inform you if you are to actually perform the tests.)

11. Explain to Gideon the preparation involved for a sigmoidoscopy. Provide him with written instructions. (Research and prepare as required.)

12. Schedule an appointment for Gideon to return for a sigmoidoscopy. (This can be performed at KMC.) Allow enough time between today's appointment and the appointment for the sigmoidoscopy to allow for preparation.

13. Explain to Gideon how to collect a stool sample and provide him with the supplies needed to do so. Ask him to return the sample to your clinic as soon as he can.

14. Dr. Greggs reviewed the results of the CBC and his white count is 11,000. Other test results indicate that Mr. Straus may indeed be anemic. Respond to the following questions in writing.

a. What is the normal white count range for an adult male?

_____

_____

_____

_____

b. Is the patient's white count within normal limits?

_____

_____

_____

_____

c. What further testing can be performed to confirm a diagnosis of anemia?

_____

_____

_____

_____

d. What other test results would need to be abnormal to indicate the possibility of anemia?

_____

_____

_____

_____

e. What are the different types of anemia?

_____

_____

_____

_____

f. What type of anemia might the patient have?

_____

_____

_____

_____

g. What would be the prognosis and treatment for anemia? (Research as needed.)

_____

_____

_____

_____

15. Perform proper hand hygiene. Properly dispose of all waste materials.

16. Record all procedures and results on a SOAP Note form and/or the patient's electronic chart. Submit all documentation to Dr. Greggs (your instructor) for review and evaluation.

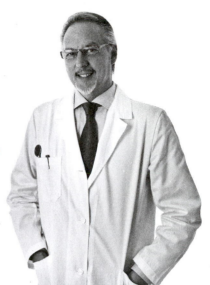

CASE STUDY **45**

Physical Examination, Immunizations, and PPD

© Minerva Studio/www.Shutterstock.com

Sally Smith has just enrolled in a medical assistant program. Before starting classes, Sally must provide documentation that she has current immunizations and a PPD test. Unfortunately Sally cannot locate her immunization records. She is at KMC today for her school physical with Dr. Bledsole. Dr. B. has decided that her best course of action would be to have a new tetanus shot, a PPD test, and her first HepB immunization, since these would satisfy the requirements for the school. Dr. B. will also be giving Sally a basic physical examination.

Respond to the following questions and perform the listed skills as ordered by Dr. Bledsole. *Skills will be accomplished by pairing with a classmate. Role-play the case study where indicated.*

1. Ms. Smith has not been seen at KMC before. Create a new patient chart (your instructor will direct whether it should be a paper or an electronic chart). If you were creating a new patient paper chart for Ms. Smith, what forms would you need to complete her file?

   _____

   _____

   _____

   _____

2. Perform medical aseptic hand hygiene and use standard precautions as appropriate.

3. Assemble equipment and supplies.

4. Introduce yourself to the patient.

5. Obtain the proper intake information.

6. Explain the procedure(s) including the risks and the normal and abnormal reactions of each injection. (Research as needed.)

7. Obtain proper consent(s).

8. Perform patient assessment including height, weight, TPR, and blood pressure. Use an oral thermometer to obtain the patient's temperature.

9. Provide the patient with instructions for proper positioning and draping in preparation for the wellness physical examination.

10. What supplies and equipment should you have available for Dr. Bledsole to complete the school physical examination?

_____

_____

_____

_____

11. Dr. Bledsole's orders are as follows:

   a. Hepatitis B vaccine—Recombivax HB 1 mL (Research the route this injection should be given: _____)

   b. Tetanus vaccine—ADACEL 0.5 mL (Research the route this injection should be given: _____)

   c. PPD test—Aplisol 0.1 mL (Research the route this injection should be given: _____)

12. Give the injections (all three injections should be given to one classmate).

13. Perform proper hand hygiene. Properly dispose of all waste materials.

14. Record all procedures and results on a SOAP Note form and/or the patient's electronic chart. Submit all documentation to Dr. Bledsole (your instructor) for review and evaluation.

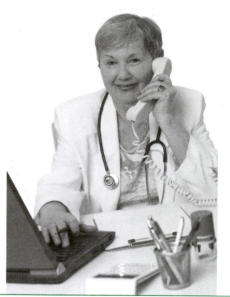

© StockLite/www.Shutterstock.com

CASE STUDY 46

Gestational Diabetes, Patient Education, and Laboratory Tests

CLINICAL

Alisa Moyer is an African American woman in her 28th week of pregnancy. Alisa is 19 years old and is pregnant for the first time. At today's visit, your physical assessment discovered that Alisa has gained 15 pounds since her last visit one month ago. Alisa claims that her dietary intake has not changed over the last month.

Dr. Carlson is concerned about gestational diabetes and has ordered an OGTT. She has asked you to explain to Alisa how to prepare for the test, which will be scheduled for tomorrow. Dr. Carlson would also like you to counsel Alisa about dietary guidelines, which should include nutrients that she and the baby need, and the restrictions that will help her to control her weight gain and to maintain her health.

Respond to the following questions and perform the listed skills as ordered by Dr. Carlson. *Skills will be accomplished by pairing with a classmate. Role-play the case study where indicated.*

1. Perform medical aseptic hand hygiene and use standard precautions as appropriate.

2. Assemble equipment and supplies. Respond in writing to the following questions: What equipment and supplies are needed for a prenatal visit? What procedures will be performed? (Research as needed.)

_____

_____

_____

_____

3. Escort Alisa to the examination room and introduce yourself.

4. Obtain and document the proper intake information.

5. Obtain the proper consent(s).

6. Perform patient assessment including height, weight, TPR, and blood pressure. Use a temporal scanner infrared thermometer to obtain the patient's temperature.

7. Collect a urine sample and process for prenatal screen. Respond in writing to the following: Why is urine tested during a prenatal appointment? What is the urine tested for? (Research as needed.)

_____

_____

_____

_____

8. Assist Dr. Carlson in a 28-week prenatal exam. Describe in writing what this might include. (Research as needed.)

_____

_____

_____

_____

9. When Dr. Carlson asks you to explain about gestational diabetes, testing, and good nutrition you discover that KMC does not have an informational pamphlet you can give to your patients. Prepare a pamphlet addressing the following topics:

- What are the main symptoms of gestational diabetes?

- What are the potential effects on the baby?

- Will gestational diabetes harm the development of the fetus?

- What risks are posed to the mother if not treated? The baby?

- What are the treatments for diabetes?

- What is the term for the acronym OGTT?

- How do you perform an OGTT?

- What preparation is involved?

- What results are healthy?

- What kind of diet restrictions would be essential?

- What is a good diet?

10. After compiling the preceding information, verbally explain the key points to Alisa.

11. Perform proper hand hygiene. Properly dispose of all waste materials.

12. Schedule an appointment for Alisa tomorrow for an OGTT.

13. Record all procedures and results on a SOAP Note form and/or the patient's electronic chart. Submit all documentation to Dr. Carlson (your instructor) for review and evaluation.

CASE STUDY 47

School Physicals, Patient Education, and Immunizations

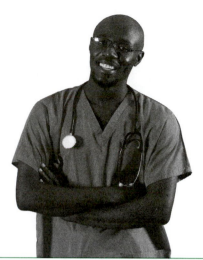

© michaeljung/www.Shutterstock.com

CLINICAL

Cruz and Nekole Saddler have brought their five-year-old twins, Nate and Tony, to KMC for the first time. Cruz and Nekole explain that they are frustrated and disagree with the requirements for school-aged children to be immunized before entry into public school. Nekole shares that their children have never had a "shot" in their lives. However, they are aware that they must comply with state regulations and have brought the children in for their kindergarten physicals. You obtain the children's vitals, perform the hearing and vision portion of the physical, and document all information.

After Bjourn performs the physical examination, he asks you to research which injections must be given in order for the children to start kindergarten. He then orders the necessary immunizations for both children and asks you to prepare and give the injections. He asks that you explain the overall purposes for immunization and the specific benefits and risks that are inherent to each immunization given to children today.

Respond to the following questions and perform the listed skills. *Skills will be accomplished by pairing with a classmate. Role-play the case study where indicated.*

1. Establish new patient charts for Nate and Tony Saddler.

2. Perform medical aseptic hand hygiene and use standard precautions as appropriate.

3. Assemble equipment and supplies.

4. Introduce yourself to the patients.

5. Obtain the proper intake information.

6. Explain the procedure(s).

7. Perform patient assessment including height, weight, TPR, and blood pressure. Use a tympanic thermometer to obtain the patients' temperatures.

8. Perform vision and hearing tests.

9. Provide the patients with instructions for proper positioning and draping in preparation for the wellness physical examination.

10. Properly position and drape the patients for the physical examination.

11. Assist Bjourn in the physical examination.

12. Perform proper hand hygiene. Properly dispose of all waste materials.

13. Record all procedures and results on a SOAP Note form and/or patients' electronic charts. Submit all documentation to Bjourn (your instructor) for review and evaluation.

14. What supplies and equipment should be made available for Bjourn to complete the physical examination? Provide the list in writing and submit it to Bjourn.

_____

_____

_____

_____

15. Respond to the following in writing: Which immunizations are required for entry into kindergarten? Are there any bioethical considerations in regard to childhood immunizations?

_____

_____

_____

_____

16. Role-play explaining the purpose of immunizations and the benefits and risks that are associated with each injection that will be given today and inform Cruz and Nekole when Nate and Tony should return for follow-up injection boosters.

17. Prepare and inject the required immunizations (your instructor will inform you as to how to proceed).

18. Submit a brief written synopsis to Bjourn of how vaccines/immunizations are stored.

19. Complete an immunization card for each patient.

20. Document all procedures in the patients' charts.

CASE STUDY 48

First Aid–Burns

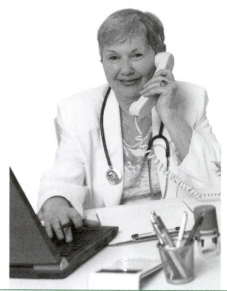

© StockLite/www.Shutterstock.com

Darlene Monson, a new patient, has come to KMC for a follow-up appointment to her emergency room visit. She was seen in the emergency room two days ago after she had dropped a basket of fries into hot oil at her place of employment. She is suffering from severe second-degree burns on her hands with some splatter burns extending toward her elbows.

You help Darlene check in and then guide her to an examination room where you obtain her vitals and conduct a patient interview about the incident and how she is feeling. You document all information in her chart and explain that Dr. Carlson will be in shortly.

Dr. Carlson would like for you to assist her in changing Darlene's bandages, during which time Dr. Carlson may examine the burns for healing and infection. There is no sign of infection and the healing process has begun. Dr. Carlson provides Darlene with instruction on how to care for her burns and writes her a prescription for pain medication.

Dr. Carlson then requests that you draft a note, for her signature, that explains that Darlene will not be returning to work until her burns completely heal. She would then like for you to schedule a follow-up appointment for Darlene and file the workers' compensation claim with Darlene's employer and the employer's insurance company.

Respond to the following questions and perform the listed skills. *Skills will be accomplished by pairing with a classmate. Role-play the case study where indicated.*

1. Establish a new patient chart.

2. Perform medical aseptic hand hygiene and use standard precautions as appropriate.

3. Assemble equipment and supplies.

4. Introduce yourself to the patient.

5. Obtain the proper intake information.

6. Explain the procedure(s).

7. Perform patient assessment including height, weight, TPR, and blood pressure. Use an oral thermometer to obtain the patient's temperature.

8. Assist in the examination of the burns as required.

9. Bandage Darlene's hands after the examination. Dr. Carlson asks you to apply burn cream on Darlene's hands before applying the bandages.

10. Provide Darlene with verbal and written instructions on caring for her burns. (Research as needed.) Create a patient pamphlet on the care of burns for future use in the clinic.

11. Prepare a prescription for Percocet 10/350 mg × 30 for Dr. Carlson's signature.

12. Write a note on the office letterhead over Dr. Carlson's signature stating that Darlene will not be returning to work until her burns have healed sufficiently, approximately 14 days.

13. Schedule an appointment for Darlene to return for a follow-up appointment in five days. Provide Darlene with an appointment reminder card.

14. Help Darlene start the workers' compensation process. Research the steps required according to your state. What forms will need to be completed? Where will the forms be submitted? What role does the clinic have in the process?

_____

_____

_____

_____

15. Perform proper hand hygiene. Properly dispose of all waste materials.

16. Record all procedures and results on a SOAP Note form and/or the patient's electronic chart. Submit all documentation to Dr. Carlson (your instructor) for review and evaluation.

CASE STUDY 49

Medication Storage

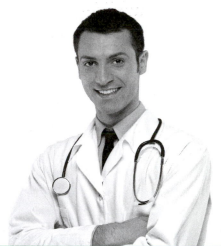

© Ljupco Smokovski/www.Shutterstock.com

CLINICAL

Dr. Greggs has been complaining about the disorganization of the medication storage room for a few weeks. He received numerous samples from a drug representative this morning and has decided that the room must be organized. He has requested that you and Jason, KMC's current extern, organize the room according to drug classifications.

You inform Jason that the medications are currently in alphabetical order and that regardless of their orientation or placement in the room, prescription safekeeping protocols must remain intact.

Respond to the following questions and perform the listed skills. *Skills will be accomplished by pairing with a classmate. Role-play the case study where indicated.*

1. Role-play with Jason, the extern, organizing the "sample" cupboard.

2. Identify and create a 3 × 5 index card with the top 50 drug classification categories. Write the category on one side of the card. On the reverse side of the card write three to five drugs that belong in the category. Place the cards in alphabetical order. Submit them to Dr. Greggs (your instructor) for approval.

3. In writing, describe prescription safekeeping protocols and submit them to Dr. Greggs.

CASE STUDY **50**

Allergy Testing

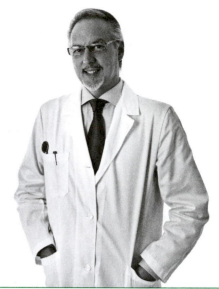

© Minerva Studio/www.Shutterstock.com

Felecia Greenbaum has an appointment today for allergy testing. Dr. Bledsole has ordered 0.1 mL of four allergens to be tested intradermally. Once it has been determined what Felecia is allergic to, weekly allergen injections will be given in the following dose schedule:

Allergenic extracts: First dose—0.01 mL
Second dose—0.02 mL
Third dose—0.03 mL

Respond to the following questions and perform the listed skills as ordered by Dr. Bledsole. *Skills will be accomplished by pairing with a classmate. Role-play the case study where indicated.*

1. Perform medical aseptic hand hygiene and use standard precautions as appropriate.

2. Assemble equipment and supplies.

3. Introduce yourself to the patient.

4. Obtain the proper intake information.

5. Explain the procedure(s), including the risks and normal and abnormal reactions. (Research as needed.)

6. Obtain the proper consent(s).

7. Perform patient assessment including height, weight, TPR, and blood pressure. Use an oral thermometer to obtain the patient's temperature.

8. Provide the patient with appropriate instructions.

9. Perform the four (4) intradermal allergy testing injections on one classmate.

10. Give the three (3) doses of the allergenic extract as ordered above. Give each injection at three different injection sites on one classmate. (Research routes

CLINICAL

109

and sites as needed.) Document in Felecia's chart, as if all injections were given in one-week progressions.

11. Perform proper hand hygiene. Properly dispose of all waste materials.

12. What emergency supplies and/or equipment will be required to be available for allergy testing and allergy injections?

_____

_____

_____

_____

13. Felecia had a severe reaction to one of the allergenic extracts. What would be the signs and symptoms and what would be your immediate response?

_____

_____

_____

_____

14. Record all procedures and results on a SOAP Note form and/or the patient's electronic chart. Submit all documentation to Dr. Bledsole (your instructor) for review and evaluation.

CASE STUDY **51**

First Aid–Bleeding

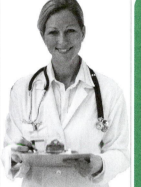

© Minerva Studio/www.Shutterstock.com

Emma Crock is a six-year-old patient who usually sees Dr. Bledsole. Emma has arrived at the clinic with a deep laceration on her right calf that is bleeding profusely. Mom, while looking a little green, is carrying Emma and is covered in blood. The towel she has wrapped around her daughter's leg is soaked through. Emma is screaming and does not want anyone to touch her "boo boo" except Dr. Bledsole, although she says maybe "the nice lady" can do it. You are not quite sure whom she is speaking of but realize that if the bleeding does not cease she may have some more serious issues develop. You approach Emma and gain her cooperation.

When you unwrap the towel from Emma's leg blood pours from the wound and for the brief moment that the wound is uncovered, before applying direct pressure, you notice that the wound is deep and about three inches in length.

Mom shares that Emma had been playing on the old rusty swing set in the backyard and caught her leg on a piece of the glider. Because they live very close to the clinic and because they are patients here, mom decided to bring Emma to the clinic instead of the hospital emergency room.

© Yuri Arcurs/www.Shutterstock.com

CLINICAL

Respond to the following questions and perform the listed skills. *Skills will be accomplished by pairing with a classmate. Role-play the case study where indicated.*

1. Perform medical aseptic hand hygiene and use standard precautions as appropriate.

2. Assemble equipment and supplies.

3. Introduce yourself to the patient. Establish a rapport with Emma to help her calm down and be distracted from her injury.

4. Obtain the proper intake information from mom.

5. Perform patient assessment including TPR. Use a tympanic thermometer to obtain the patient's temperature.

6. Dr. Bledsole is in with another patient, but after you inform him of the situation he comes with you to see Emma. Dr. Bledsole asks you to first elevate the leg, and apply pressure to the appropriate pressure point. Dr. Bledsole takes over

holding pressure and asks you to find Chris Taylor (the PA) or one of the nurses or another medical assistant to come in and help. Chandra, one of the medical assistants comes, and Dr. Bledsole has her take over applying pressure while you set up the room for a surgical repair of the laceration. While collecting supplies you see Chris and ask her to go to Emma's examination room as well.

7. Answer the following in writing: What supplies and equipment will be required for a surgical repair of a laceration?

   _____

   _____

   _____

   _____

8. Physically set up the room for Dr. Bledsole's inspection.

9. Emma is not doing well. She is very pale, her respirations are rapid, and she is vomiting. However, the bleeding has slowed down as long as pressure is applied to the pressure point. Chris starts an IV in the back of Emma's left hand.

10. Dr. Bledsole orders a one-time dose of ketamine 0.4 mg/kg IM and atropine 0.01 mg/kg IM and asks you to prepare and then give the injection to Emma. Emma weighs 50 pounds.

11. Open the sterile packs and other supplies needed for the repair, then perform a surgical scrub and drape the area.

12. Dr. Bledsole requests 1% lidocaine with epinephrine in amounts to achieve anesthesia. He also requests 4.0 absorbable suture for deep repair and 5.0 Prolene suture for superficial repairs.

13. Assist Dr. Bledsole and Chris as required during the repair.

14. Monitor Emma's pulse and respiration throughout the procedure.

15. Once Dr. Bledsole has finished suturing Emma's leg, he requests that you apply dressings and provide mom with instructions on how to care for the wound. Be sure to include instructions on watching for infection. Emma should return to the clinic immediately if signs of infection occur. Emma's immunization records are reviewed and she is current on her tetanus.

16. Emma's mom should be instructed to give Emma Tylenol and ibuprofen alternately as needed for pain.

17. Record all procedures and results on a SOAP Note form and/or the patient's electronic chart. Submit all documentation to Dr. Bledsole (your instructor) for review and evaluation.

18. Perform proper hand hygiene.

19. Clean the room. Properly dispose of all waste materials.

20. Prepare the surgical packs for sterilization and replace equipment and supplies as needed.

CASE STUDY **52**

Hypertensive Emergency

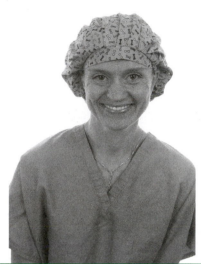

CLINICAL

Arthur and Desiree Hensley have arrived at the clinic. Arthur, a 37-year-old patient, was seen two weeks ago and was diagnosed with Stage 2 hypertension. Dr. Wertz put him on medication to lower his blood pressure. She spoke with him about dietary changes and an exercise program that would also help him.

Desiree is leading Arthur slowly by the arm and is speaking for him. You notice that Arthur seems to be very confused about his surroundings and that he seems to be experiencing shortness of breath (SOB). You immediately help him into a wheelchair and escort the Hensleys into an examination room. Once there, you perform Arthur's vitals and find that his blood pressure is 178/118 mm Hg. Desiree is very worried and does not know if Arthur has been taking his medication as directed. She states that he has been complaining of a headache for two days and that today he has been "in and out of it."

You explain to Arthur and Desiree that Dr. Wertz may want to run some tests and that she will be in very soon. You then help Arthur onto the examination table and provide him with a gown.

Dr. Wertz examines Arthur and asks you to perform an ECG. You do this and give Dr. Wertz the prepared strips. Dr. Wertz tells you to call for an ambulance and then explain to the Hensleys that Arthur is experiencing a hypertensive emergency and needs to be transferred to the hospital immediately.

Respond to the following questions and perform the listed skills as ordered by Dr. Wertz. *Skills will be accomplished by pairing with a classmate. Role-play the case study where indicated.*

1. Identify the patient and introduce yourself.

2. Escort Mr. Hensley to the examination room via wheelchair.

3. Perform medical aseptic hand hygiene and use standard precautions as appropriate.

4. Assemble equipment and supplies.

5. Obtain and document the proper intake information.

6. Obtain the proper consent(s).

7. Perform patient assessment including height, weight, TPR, and blood pressure. Use an oral thermometer to obtain the patient's temperature.

8. Arthur's BP reading is high; notify Dr. Wertz immediately.

9. Dr. Wertz requests that you start Mr. Hensley on two liters of oxygen by cannula.

10. Explain to the Hensleys that Dr. Wertz has ordered some tests and that she will be in very soon to examine Arthur.

11. Provide Arthur with a gown or drape and ask him to disrobe appropriately for the examination being performed.

12. Assist Dr. Wertz in the procedure(s) as needed.

13. Dr. Wertz orders an ECG.

14. Perform the ECG and give the results to Dr. Wertz for interpretation.

15. Dr. Wertz asks you to call for an ambulance immediately.

16. Explain to the Hensleys that Arthur is experiencing a hypertensive emergency and needs to be transported to the hospital immediately.

17. Prepare Mr. Hensley to be transported. (Provide the paramedics with a copy of the SOAP Notes and a copy of the ECG.)

18. Research and write a two-paragraph informational report on hypertensive emergencies. Submit it to Dr. Wertz (your instructor).

CASE STUDY **53**

Choking, Pediatric

You are in the process of checking in a patient who has just arrived at the clinic for an appointment. Just as you are reaching for his insurance card, you see a small child approximately four years old and 30 pounds in the waiting room who appears to be actively choking and in distress. The mother does not appear to know that her child is choking because she is focused on filling out a new patient packet.

Respond to the following questions and perform the listed skills. *Skills will be accomplished by pairing with a classmate. Role-play the case study where indicated.*

1. Role-play the scenario. As part of the role-play you must assess the situation and identify the necessary steps in providing emergency care to the child. (If necessary, research before participating in the role-play.)

2. Demonstrate the ability to perform abdominal thrusts on a small child.

3. Respond to the following in writing:

   a. Are there any contraindications to performing abdominal thrusts? If so, list and describe them.

   _____

   _____

   _____

   _____

   b. Describe the differences in performing abdominal thrusts on an infant, a child, and an adult.

   _____

   _____

   _____

   _____

CLINICAL

c. Describe the appropriate response had the abdominal thrusts not been successful.

_____

_____

_____

_____

4. Document all information on a SOAP Note form and/or the patient's electronic medical records (to be filed in the mother's medical record).

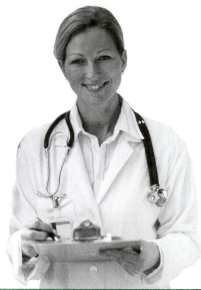

© Yuri Arcurs/www.Shutterstock.com

CASE STUDY 54

Respiratory Distress

Peter Cooper, an established patient, has arrived for his scheduled appointment with Chris Taylor. Peter is blind and requires extra care when maneuvering around the office. You guide Peter to an examination room and obtain his vitals. You notice that Peter seems to be coughing quite a bit and is having trouble breathing. You ask Peter the necessary information about his symptoms and document them in his chart.

Chris has two patients in front of Mr. Cooper; this prompts your decision to discuss the situation with Chris as she is readying to enter another patient's examination room. Chris would like for you to test Mr. Cooper's pulmonary functions by first doing a pulse oximetry and then a spirometry test. You provide Chris with the results, and after attending to Mr. Cooper, Chris requests that you provide Mr. Cooper with a nebulizer treatment and schedule him for a chest X-ray to test for pneumonia.

Respond to the following questions and perform the listed skills. *Skills will be accomplished by pairing with a classmate. Role-play the case study where indicated.*

1. Perform medical aseptic hand hygiene and use standard precautions as appropriate.

2. Assemble equipment and supplies.

3. Introduce yourself to the patient.

4. Obtain the proper intake information.

5. Explain the procedure(s).

6. Perform patient assessment including height, weight, TPR, and blood pressure. Use a temporal scanner infrared thermometer to obtain the patient's temperature.

7. Perform the pulse oximetry. Mr. Cooper's results are a little low but are WNL. What are normal limits for pulse oximetry?

_____

_____

_____

_____

8. Perform a spirometry test. All of Mr. Cooper's results are WNL. What are the normal limits for spirometry testing?

_____

_____

_____

_____

9. Prepare and administer a nebulizer treatment for Mr. Cooper.

10. Call the clinic's laboratory and schedule a chest X-ray. Walk Mr. Cooper down to the laboratory.

11. Chris reviews the chest X-ray with Dr. Bledsole, and they determine that Mr. Cooper does indeed have pneumonia.

12. Chris and Dr. Bledsole would like to hospitalize Mr. Cooper for a couple of days to start him on IV antibiotics.

13. Role-play calling the hospital to have Mr. Cooper admitted.

14. Collect all of the necessary information required to admit Mr. Cooper. (Research as necessary.)

15. Perform proper hand hygiene. Properly dispose of all waste materials.

16. Record all procedures and results on a SOAP Note form and/or the patient's electronic chart. Submit all documentation to Chris (your instructor) for review and evaluation.

17. Mr. Cooper has Mailhandlers as his primary insurance. Complete a claim form to be mailed to Mr. Cooper's insurance company. (Create Mr. Cooper's information.)

DX: R/O Pneumonia
Procedures: Established patient—Office visit
                Pulse oximetry
                Spirometry
                Nebulizer

CASE STUDY 55

Electrocardiography, Venipuncture

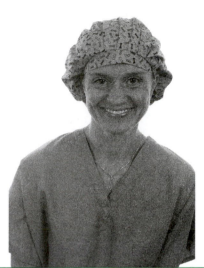

© rj lerich/www.Shutterstock.com

Millicent St. Vincent (Mrs.), a 67-year-old patient of Dr. Wertz, lives two blocks from the clinic. She called the clinic 10 minutes ago, complaining of chest pain. She stated that it started just after lunch. The pain began as tightness in her chest but she has now developed a sharp pain that goes through to her back and into her shoulder. She denied any shortness of breath or diaphoresis, although she does have some mild nausea. The receptionist told her to come right in and the clinic would work her in.

When Mrs. St. Vincent arrives, you immediately take her to an examination room, obtain her vital signs, and ask her the standard questions. She is visibly agitated and is exhibiting obvious signs of pain in her chest. She tells you that she had a Polish hotdog with sauerkraut and french fries for lunch. She has taken two antacids, but they did not help. She denies the use of alcohol, drugs, or tobacco products. She has a family history of cancer, diabetes, myocardial infarction, hypercholesterolemia, hypertension, stroke, and CHF. Mrs. St. Vincent exercises <3×/week. She weighs 134 lb. 0 oz.; height 5'6"; temperature 97.4; pulse: 80; pulse OX: 97; BP: 125/80; and has no known allergies.

You ask Mrs. St. Vincent to disrobe to her waist and provide her with a gown, asking her to tie it in the front. You then tell her that Dr. Wertz with be right in.

The following is Dr. Wertz's findings after the examination.

PHYSICAL FINDINGS: The patient is an appropriately alert, well-nourished, well-developed female. HEENT: PERRLA, sclera clear; Throat: Intact gag reflex; Neck: Supple no adenopathy. No carotid bruits. Lungs: Clear to auscultation, breath sounds equal. CV: RRR no murmurs, gallops, or rubs. Skin: Warm and dry; there is no rash, diaphoresis, or mottling. Lower extremities: No edema.

Dr. Wertz orders the following tests: ECG, CBC, CK, CK-MB, and Troponin.

Respond to the following questions and perform the listed skills as ordered by Dr. Wertz. *Skills will be accomplished by pairing with a classmate. Role-play the case study where indicated.*

1. Mrs. St. Vincent is an existing patient and will not require a new patient chart.

2. Perform medical aseptic hand hygiene and use standard precautions as appropriate.

3. Assemble equipment and supplies.

4. Introduce yourself to the patient.

5. Obtain the proper intake information.

6. Explain the procedure(s).

7. Obtain the proper consent(s).

8. Perform patient assessment including height, weight, TPR, and blood pressure. Use a temporal scanner infrared thermometer to take her temperature.

9. Ask Mrs. St Vincent to disrobe and provide her with a gown.

10. Perform an ECG.

11. Depending on the type of ECG machine your clinic has, either mount and provide appropriate patient information on the mounted ECG or print out the ECG tracing.

12. Ask Mrs. St. Vincent to dress.

13. Perform venipuncture.

14. Draw the correct number and color-topped tubes for each test ordered. (Research as needed.)

15. Perform proper hand hygiene. Properly dispose of all waste materials.

16. Package specimens to be sent to the laboratory for testing.

17. Explain why CK, CK-MB, and troponin tests are ordered and how their results help in determining a diagnosis. (Research as needed.)

_____

_____

_____

_____

18. Identify the medical terms associated with the following abbreviations.

   a. CHF: _____

   b. <3×/week: _____

   c. HEENT: _____

   d. PERRLA: _____

   e. CV: _____

   f. RRR: _____

   g. ECG: _____

   h. CBC: _____

   i. CK: _____

19. Identify the possibly fatal error the receptionist made.

_____

_____

_____

_____

20. Record all procedures and results on a SOAP Note form and/or the patient's electronic chart. Submit all documentation to Dr. Wertz (your instructor) for review and evaluation.

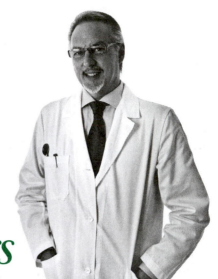

© Minerva Studio/www.Shutterstock.com

CASE STUDY 56

Urinalysis, Catheterization, and Communication Barriers

Sonia Mendez is a 30-year-old new patient who does not speak English. Her cousin Rose has brought Sonia to the clinic today. Through translation, performed by Rose, you find that Sonia has been complaining of voiding only a very little amount of urine but feels as if her bladder is distended and full. Sonia has been drinking six large glasses of water for the last two days in the hope of making more urine. Upon further questioning it is revealed that Sonia had a laparoscopy and D&C performed by a Dr. Emanuel Gonzales (who is not employed by KMC) two days ago, and since then she has not been able to urinate correctly.

You speak with Dr. Bledsole, who orders a CBC with ESR, BUN, creatinine level, Foley catheterization, and urinalysis to verify that her bladder and kidneys are working and that there is no infection present.

Respond to the following questions and perform the listed skills as ordered by Dr. Bledsole. *Skills will be accomplished by pairing with a classmate. Role-play the case study where indicated.*

1. Ms. Mendez is a new patient to KMC and will require a new patient chart. You will also need to request her records from Dr. Gonzales. Complete the required consent forms, and appropriately fax them to Dr. Gonzales's office.

2. Perform medical aseptic hand hygiene and use standard precautions as appropriate.

3. Assemble equipment and supplies. Respond in writing to the following question: What equipment and supplies are needed for these procedures?

   _____

   _____

   _____

   _____

CLINICAL

4. Escort Sonia and Rose to the examination room and introduce yourself. (Role-play steps 4–8 with classmates, keeping in mind that Sonia does not speak English and that Rose is translating.)

5. Obtain and document the proper intake information.

6. Obtain the proper consent(s).

7. Perform patient assessment including height, weight, TPR, and blood pressure. Use a tympanic thermometer to obtain the patient's temperature. Sonia's temperature is 101.8°F. Why would her temperature be elevated?

_____

_____

_____

_____

8. Perform a venipuncture, collecting the correct number and color-topped tubes for the requested laboratory tests. Send the specimens to the laboratory for processing. Identify the correct order of draw for the evacuated tubes. (Note: Your instructor will inform you if you are to perform these laboratory tests.)

9. Provide Sonia with a gown or drape and ask her to disrobe.

10. Explain how a Foley catheterization works. Explain to Sonia how she will be positioned and how the gown and drape should be placed. Respond in writing and address during the role-play.

11. Assist Dr. Bledsole in the procedure, as needed.

12. The catheter released 1,000 milliliters of urine. (Convert milliliters into liters for charting purposes. Research as necessary.)

13. Perform a full urinalysis on the urine collected. Briefly describe, in writing, the sequence of events for a full urinalysis.

14. Dr. Bledsole reviews the results of the CBC with ESR, BUN, creatinine levels, and the UA and, based on the results and under the circumstances of Sonia's recent surgery, orders a catheter leg bag to be placed on Sonia for three days. This will aid her bladder to start working properly again. Explain to Sonia the need for the procedure and how it is performed. Include information on how to empty the bag and ask her to keep track of the amount of urine in the bag before emptying it.

15. Dr. Bledsole also orders Furadantin 100 mg q.i.d. for seven days. Write a prescription for Dr. Bledsole's signature.

16. Assemble all necessary equipment and supplies.

17. Assist Dr. Bledsole in the procedure, as needed.

18. Perform proper hand hygiene. Properly dispose of all waste materials.

19. Inform Sonia about what to expect regarding any symptoms she may experience from the procedures. Instruct her as to when to return to the clinic to have the catheter removed.

20. Record all procedures and results on a SOAP Note form and/or the patient's electronic chart. Submit all documentation to Dr. Bledsole (your instructor) for review and evaluation.

CASE STUDY 57

Fracture

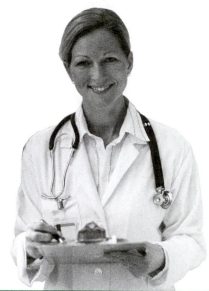

Michael Evans is an 11-year-old boy who has been a patient at KMC since birth. Michael is very active in sports and enjoys hiking and running the most. Michael had been hiking with the Boy Scouts this morning and had been running in the mountains when he fell to the ground screaming that he was in "massive pain" and that his left leg is "killing him."

The scout leader rushed Michael down the mountain and telephoned his aunt on the way to the clinic. Michael has been staying with his aunt for the summer while his parents travel. The scout leader carried Michael into the clinic with his aunt following behind. You can visibly see the distress and pain that Michael is feeling. When you performed the patient assessment you noted that Michael has grown over six inches since his last physical examination, almost one year ago. You document the information and help Michael into a wheelchair and take him back to an examination room.

When Chris Taylor, PA, examines Michael, she observes that his left femur is definitely swollen and is not properly aligned. Chris orders an AP, lateral, and PA X-ray of Michael's leg. After examining the X-rays Chris suspects a nondisplaced femur fracture at the growth plate and suggests that Michael be scheduled for an appointment with an orthopedic surgeon as soon as possible.

Chris will apply a full leg, non-weight-bearing gutter cast. She has requested that you call Dr. Walkerton's office, an orthopedic surgeon, and schedule an appointment for Michael within the next two days. Chris would like for you to measure Michael for crutches and help him become familiar with using them. She would also like for you to explain to Michael how to care for his cast.

Chris has ordered Demerol 45 mg IM to be given to Michael before he leaves the clinic. Demerol is supplied 50 mg/5 mL.

Chris wants you to write a prescription for #20, 5 mg Lortab, q4h, PRN pain, for her signature.

Respond to the following questions and perform the listed skills as ordered by Chris Taylor. *Skills will be accomplished by pairing with a classmate. Role-play the case study where indicated.*

1. Michael is an existing patient and will not require a new patient chart.

2. Answer the following questions in writing:

   a. Can Chris legally treat Michael without his parents' permission? Describe the considerations and processes for both yes and no responses.

   b. What is the normal rate of growth for an 11-year-old boy?

   c. Could growing over six inches during the past year affect the femur break? Defend your response.

   d. What kind of nonverbal communication, displayed by Michael, would leave you to believe that he is experiencing distress and pain? What question(s) will you ask regarding pain during the patient assessment?

3. Perform medical aseptic hand hygiene and use standard precautions as appropriate.

4. Assemble equipment and supplies.

5. Introduce yourself to the patient.

6. Obtain the proper intake information.

7. Obtain proper consents.

8. Perform patient assessment including height, weight, TPR, and blood pressure. Use a tympanic thermometer to obtain the patient's temperature.

9. Explain the procedure and take Michael to be X-rayed. Role-play performing the X-rays (with or without X-ray equipment available in your school). Respond in writing to the following: Identify and explain the different types of fractures that can occur in the femur. What is the name of the fracture that typically occurs at the growth plate?

   _____

   _____

   _____

   _____

10. Assemble supplies and equipment for a full-leg gutter cast. (Research as needed.)

11. Assist Chris, as needed, with the application of the cast.

12. Measure Michael for crutches. Explain crutch use and cast care. Be sure to emphasize that it is critical that Michael is non-weight bearing.

13. Prepare and administer Demerol injection.

14. Prepare the requested prescription for Chris's signature.

15. Perform proper hand hygiene. Properly dispose of all waste materials.

16. Call Dr. Walkerton's office and schedule an appointment for tomorrow, if possible.

17. Inform Michael and his aunt of his scheduled appointment with Dr. Walkerton.

18. Record all procedures and results on a SOAP Note form and/or the patient's electronic chart. Submit all documentation to Chris (your instructor) for review and evaluation.

CASE STUDY 58

Specialty Examination, Sigmoidoscopy

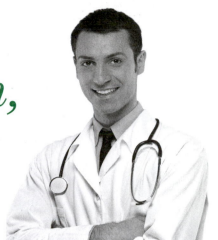

© Ljupco Smokovski/www.Shutterstock.com

Gideon Straus will be in for his scheduled sigmoidoscopy today. Dr. Greggs would like for you to prepare the room, assist with the procedure, explain the benefits of a more fibrous diet, and schedule a follow-up appointment.

Gideon is also returning his guaiac test card. Dr. Greggs would like for you to process the specimen and report the results to him immediately.

Respond to the following questions and perform the listed skills as ordered by Dr. Greggs. *Skills will be accomplished by pairing with a classmate. Role-play the case study where indicated.*

1. Perform medical aseptic hand hygiene and use standard precautions as appropriate.

2. Assemble equipment and supplies.

3. Prepare the room for the procedure.

4. Introduce yourself to the patient.

5. Obtain the proper intake information. Ensure that Gideon has followed the necessary preparation for the procedure.

6. Obtain proper consents.

7. Perform patient assessment including height, weight, TPR, and blood pressure. Use a tympanic thermometer to obtain the patient's temperature.

8. Process the guaiac test and provide Dr. Greggs with the results. (Note: Your instructor will inform you if you are to actually perform the tests.)

9. Explain the procedure.

10. Explain disrobing, gowning, draping, and positioning for this procedure.

11. Assist Dr. Greggs, as needed, with the sigmoidoscopy.

12. Label the specimens and process to send to the laboratory.

13. Explain to the patient the benefits of a more fibrous diet. Respond in writing to the following question: How would a more fibrous diet be helpful to Gideon? In order to add more fiber, what changes could he make to his existing diet?

14. Perform proper hand hygiene. Properly dispose of all waste materials.

15. Schedule a follow-up appointment for Gideon and provide him with the time and date of the appointment.

16. Record all procedures and results on a SOAP Note form and then input the information into the medical software data bank in the patient's electronic chart. Submit all documentation to Chris (your instructor) for review and evaluation.

CASE STUDY 59

Endocrine Disorder

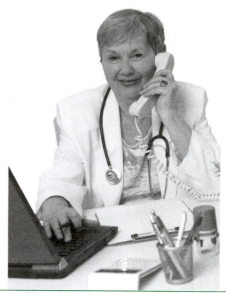

Rain Story is a 24-year-old woman who has arrived at the clinic for the appointment that was scheduled for her with Dr. Carlson. You escort Ms. Story to an examination room and proceed to obtain her history. Rain informs you that she is about 6 weeks pregnant and that she miscarried at about 12 weeks last year. She has been feeling "very sluggish," is "always freezing," has "horrible headaches," and has been experiencing muscle cramping. She is very worried about her baby and her body. You document all of this information in Ms. Story's chart.

You explain to Ms. Story that Dr. Carlson will want to check her and the baby to see how they are both doing. You provide Ms. Story with a gown and sheet and explain how to use them. You will assist Dr. Carlson with the examination.

Dr. Carlson would like for you to perform a venipuncture on Ms. Story. She would like for you to run a CBC and to draw tubes for an hCG to determine the progress of the pregnancy and a TSH test to check for hypothyroidism. These are to be sent to the laboratory. Standard office procedure requires you to collect a clean-catch urine sample on all pregnant women and perform a UA physical and chemical examination and run a pregnancy test.

After completing the physical examination and reviewing the test results, Dr. Carlson requests that you schedule an appointment for Ms. Story with an endocrinologist.

Respond to the following questions and perform the listed skills as ordered by Dr. Carlson. *Skills will be accomplished by pairing with a classmate. Role-play the case study where indicated.*

1. Create a new patient chart.

2. Perform medical aseptic hand hygiene and use standard precautions as appropriate.

CLINICAL

133

3. Assemble equipment and supplies. Respond in writing to the following question: What equipment and supplies are needed for these procedures? (Research as necessary.)

_____

_____

_____

_____

4. Escort Ms. Story to the examination room and introduce yourself.

5. Obtain and document the proper intake information.

6. Obtain proper consents.

7. Perform patient assessment including height, weight, TPR, and blood pressure. Use a tympanic thermometer to obtain the patient's temperature.

8. Obtain a clean-catch urine sample. Explain the procedure to the patient.

9. Perform a pregnancy test and a UA physical and chemical examination.

10. Explain a prenatal examination to Ms. Story. (Research as needed.)

11. Ask Ms. Story to disrobe and provide her with a gown and drape.

12. Explain to Ms. Story how she should be positioned and how the gown and drape should be placed.

13. Assist the physician in the procedure as required.

14. Perform proper hand hygiene. Properly dispose of all waste materials.

15. Inform Ms. Story that she can get dressed and that you will be drawing some blood for tests that Dr. Carlson has ordered. Explain to her when she may expect the results.

16. Perform a venipuncture.

17. Draw the correct number and color-topped tubes for each test ordered during the role-play. (Research as needed.)

18. Would Dr. Carlson order a quantitative or qualitative hCG blood test? Explain your answer.

_____

_____

_____

_____

19. Perform proper hand hygiene. Properly dispose of all waste materials.

20. Package the specimens to be sent to the laboratory for testing.

21. Explain why CBC and TSH tests are ordered and how their results help in determining a diagnosis. (Research as needed.) Submit it, in writing, to your instructor for evaluation.

22. Record all procedures on a SOAP Note form and/or the patient's electronic chart. Submit all documentation to Dr. Carlson (your instructor) for review and evaluation.

23. Schedule an appointment for Ms. Story with an endocrinologist. Provide Ms. Story with a referral card or make the call yourself by role-playing with a classmate.

24. Research as needed and respond to the following questions (submit your answers to your instructor):

    a. Why did Dr. Carlson suspect a thyroid problem?

    _____

    _____

    _____

    _____

    b. What is the percentage of a miscarriage to a woman who has hypothyroidism?

    _____

    _____

    _____

    _____

CASE STUDY 60

Prescription Drug Abuse, Patient Advocate

Adam Hutchins is an established patient and is still under care for herniated discs in his neck that occurred during a car accident approximately six months ago. He was in the clinic two weeks ago for a refill of muscle relaxants and pain pills. During that visit, he revealed that someone had stolen his medication and that he "really" needed a refill. Dr. Bledsole wrote a prescription for a one-month supply with the understanding that this was a one-time occurrence and that Adam was to be seen by a pain management specialist for further prescriptions.

Today, Adam is in visible pain and offers up another explanation as to why he no longer has medications available for pain relief. He explains that he cannot be seen at the pain clinic until the end of next week and "just needs a two-week refill."

You suspect that Adam is misusing his medications and proceed to inform Dr. Bledsole, who, after speaking with Adam, agrees with your assessment. Dr. Bledsole would like for you to act as a patient advocate for Adam and to provide him with a list of resources where he may obtain help and information on misusing medications.

Respond to the following questions and perform the listed skills. *Skills will be accomplished by pairing with a classmate. Role-play the case study where indicated.* You may be asked to work in pairs on this project as indicated by your instructor.

1. Perform medical aseptic hand hygiene and use standard precautions as appropriate.

2. Escort Adam to an examination room and introduce yourself.

3. Obtain and document the proper intake information.

4. Perform patient assessment including height, weight, TPR, and blood pressure. Use a tympanic thermometer to obtain the patient's temperature.

5. Prepare the patient for examination by Dr. Bledsole. After examining Adam, Dr. Bledsole asks you to provide Adam with information on substance abuse and to document all information in Adam's chart.

6. Why do you think that Adam is misusing his medications? What communication skills were necessary in determining your response? Respond to the questions in writing and make a list of the examples that led you to believe that Adam is misusing.

7. Are you required to report substance abuse to any agency? If so, what agency or agencies?

_____

_____

_____

_____

8. How would you document suspected misuse of medication in Adam's chart? Provide the response in writing as if documenting in the patient's chart.

9. Research available resources in your area that you can provide to Adam for his substance abuse. Provide these resources in writing to Dr. Bledsole (your instructor).

10. Research the following information and role-play being a patient advocate with a classmate, with you acting as the medical assistant and the classmate as Adam. Reverse roles.

    • What is prescription medication substance abuse?

    • What are the indications of an abuser?

    • What are some commonly abused prescription medications?

    • What potential issues may arise if an abuser does not receive treatment?

    • What are the pain management resources available in your area?

    • What are the substance abuse resources available in your area?

11. Create a patient information pamphlet for future use at KMC regarding substance abuse and address the topics that you researched for step 10. Submit this pamphlet to Dr. Bledsole (your instructor).

CASE STUDY 61

Possible Spousal Abuse Emergency Triage

John Ardell accompanied his wife Stacy to the clinic today seeking a walk-in appointment. He explains that Stacy slipped and fell on some ice while walking to her car last night. John tells you that aside from some cuts and bruises on her body, her "arm socket" is really hurting her. He states that "she may need an X-ray" and some "drugs" to help her with the pain.

You notice that Stacy is consistently looking away from you as her husband talks. She seems very tense and anxious. You make the decision, after looking at the schedule, that Stacy can be seen in about 20 minutes. You inform John and Stacy and ask them to take a seat in the waiting room.

You are going to perform the necessary triage and vital signs on Stacy and call her name in the waiting room. John immediately stands up to escort Stacy. You inform John that there is no room available at this time and that you are going to bring Stacy back to the waiting room after you obtain her vital signs and some other basic information. John becomes irate and demands to be present with Stacy to "provide her with support." Stacy then becomes physically stressed and upset.

Respond to the following questions and perform the listed skills. *Skills will be accomplished by pairing with a classmate. Role-play the case study where indicated.*

1. Role-play the opening situation. Greet the patient and her spouse, and after listening to their situation, ask them to have a seat in the waiting area.

2. Do you feel that Stacy has been abused? Why or why not? Do you need to inform anyone of your suspicions? If so, who? If not, why not? Defend your response in writing.

3. Does this patient require an appointment preference for suspected safety measures? Explain and defend your response in writing.

4. Describe in writing the verbal and nonverbal communication involved with this patient and her spouse.

5. Describe in writing the type of communication skills that you will need to employ to appropriately handle this type of situation.

COMPREHENSIVE

6. Continue to role-play the scenario.

7. Describe in writing why you handled the situation as you did and what you think may happen next.

8. Are there any legal or ethical implications involved with this scenario? (Research as needed.) If so, what are they? Do you think they are necessary and effective? If not, should some be established? What type of implications should there be? Defend your response in a one-page informative or argumentative paper. Your paper should be free of errors (grammatical, sentence structure, punctuation, and information).

9. Submit all responses to your instructor.

CASE STUDY **62**

Walk-In Emergency, Triage, and Follow-Up

John Ardell, Stacy Ardell's husband, has been asked to leave the clinic after becoming angry and defensive. Stacy has stayed to receive care for injuries that were reported to have been caused by her slipping on ice last night. Stacy has been escorted to an examination room and has been informed of her rights as a patient.

Chris Taylor, PA, has asked you to obtain Stacy's vital signs and any information about the occurrence that Stacy is willing to share. When you began questioning Stacy about her injuries, she becomes quiet and will only agree with what her husband has stated about the incident. You decide to ask Stacy about the accident with different types of questions. Stacy relents and begins to tell you what has really happened.

You document and inform Chris of the information obtained from Stacy. Chris performs a physical examination on Stacy. She asks you to prepare Stacy for an X-ray and to obtain one of Stacy's shoulder. The X-ray reveals a dislocation of the humerus and the scapula. Chris has recommended that Stacy be taken to the hospital for treatment and that the hospital be made aware of the situation. She would like for you to act as a patient advocate to Stacy while she is waiting for transportation to the hospital.

Respond to the following questions and perform the listed skills. *Skills will be accomplished by pairing with a classmate. Role-play the case study where indicated.*

1. Identify the patient and introduce yourself.

2. Escort Stacy back to an examination room.

3. Perform medical aseptic hand hygiene and use standard precautions as appropriate.

4. Perform patient assessment including height, weight, TPR, and blood pressure. Use an oral thermometer to obtain the patient's temperature.

5. Interview Stacy. Provide your instructor with a two-paragraph overview of your interview with Stacy and describe why you asked the questions that you did. How many different ways/tactics did it take for Stacy to share her story?

COMPREHENSIVE

141

6. Prepare Stacy for a physical examination. Provide her with a gown and explain the procedure.

7. Assist Chris with the procedure.

8. Your instructor will direct you in how to proceed with the X-ray. Some states do not allow medical assistants to perform X-rays, in which case "obtaining an X-ray" may involve escorting Stacy to the radiology department, or you may be asked to describe the process in writing.

9. Call for transportation to the hospital emergency department for Stacy.

10. Act as a patient advocate. Describe in writing what this means and what you would do in this role.

11. Document all procedures.

12. Dispose of examination room materials as appropriate and perform proper hand hygiene.

13. Submit all responses and documentation to Chris (your instructor) for review and evaluation.

CASE STUDY **63**

Type 1 Diabetes, Laboratory Tests

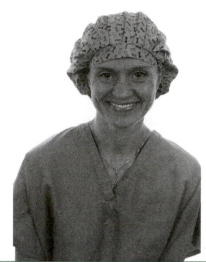

Austin Garcia is a 16-year-old male patient of Dr. Wertz. Austin's mother has brought him today because Austin has been complaining of always being thirsty and hungry and gets lightheaded if he does not eat. Austin also tells you that "it seems like I always have to pee." You take Austin back to an examination room and perform a patient assessment. After visiting with Austin, Dr. Wertz orders a urinalysis and blood glucose POCT. His blood glucose levels are high in both tests. Dr. Wertz then orders a fasting blood sugar (FBS) test and an HbA1c for the following day.

Austin's mom brings him to the clinic the next day and after determining that your instructions have been followed, you start the three-hour FBS. Austin is feeling very shaky and lightheaded. After the second blood draw you notice he is trembling and seems very confused. You take the appropriate actions. Dr. Wertz comes to the examination room and immediately starts an IV glucose infusion. Austin returns to a normal state almost immediately.

After this episode Dr. Wertz diagnoses Austin with type 1 diabetes. She would like to have it confirmed by having Austin go to the hospital for a GTT as soon as possible. You will need to schedule this test for Austin.

Respond to the following questions and perform the listed skills as ordered by Dr. Wertz. *Skills will be accomplished by pairing with a classmate. Role-play the case study where indicated.*

1. Austin is an existing patient and will not require a new patient chart.

2. Perform medical aseptic hand hygiene and use standard precautions as appropriate.

3. Assemble equipment and supplies.

4. Introduce yourself to the patient.

5. Obtain the proper intake information.

6. Explain the procedure(s).

7. Perform patient assessment including height, weight, TPR, and blood pressure. Use a temporal scanner infrared thermometer to obtain the patient's temperature.

8. Perform a UA dip. Austin's blood glucose results are high. (Record classmates' results and then record a "high" reading for Austin's blood glucose results in parentheses.) What is the normal blood glucose range for a UA blood sugar?

_____

_____

_____

_____

9. Perform a capillary stick and POCT blood glucose. Austin's blood glucose results are high. (Record classmates' results and then record a "high" reading for Austin's blood glucose results in parentheses.) What is the normal blood glucose range for a POCT blood glucose test?

_____

_____

_____

_____

10. Verbally describe the procedure and preparation for a three-hour FBS to a classmate and document the patient instructions on a SOAP Note form for Austin's file or in the patient's electronic chart.

11. Perform a three-hour FBS. To accommodate a classroom setting, perform the blood draws in the correctly colored top tube 45 minutes apart. (Note: You will only perform two draws on the same patient because the third draw will not be done due to Austin's reaction to the test.)

12. Perform an HbA1c as a Point-of-Care test.

13. Once Austin (classmate should role-play this situation) begins to get lightheaded, gets confused, and is trembling, what would be your appropriate course of action?

_____

_____

_____

_____

14. Why did Austin return to normal after Dr. Wertz started the IV glucose infusion?

_____

_____

_____

_____

15. What are the correct medical terms for:

a. Excessive thirst: _____

b. Excessive eating: _____

c. Excessive urination: _____

d. Excessive sugar in the blood: _____

16. Schedule the GTT with the hospital. What patient information will you need to schedule this outpatient test? (Verbally record scheduling the GTT for Dr. Wertz's review and evaluation.)

_____

_____

_____

_____

17. Perform proper hand hygiene. Properly dispose of all waste materials.

18. Record all procedures and results on a SOAP Note form and/or the patient's electronic chart. Submit all documentation to Dr. Wertz (your instructor) for review and evaluation.

CASE STUDY **64**

Insurance Billing and Coding, Laboratory Tests

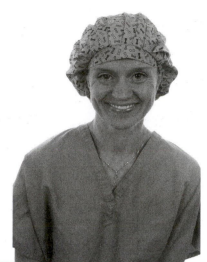

Austin Garcia is a 16-year-old male existing patient of Dr. Wertz. Austin's mother brought him in yesterday complaining of always being thirsty and hungry and gets lightheaded if he does not eat. Austin also stated that "it seems like I always have to pee." Dr. Wertz spent 30 minutes evaluating Austin and then ordered a UA dipstick and blood glucose POCT. Dr. Wertz diagnosed Austin with type 1 diabetes but has ordered a fasting blood sugar (FBS) test and an HbA1C to confirm the diagnosis for today.

Today during the FBS Austin began to feel very shaky and lightheaded. After the second blood draw he began trembling and seemed very confused. Dr. Wertz immediately started an IV glucose infusion. Austin returned to a normal state almost immediately. (See Case Study 63.)

After receiving the results of the FBS and HbA1c lab tests Dr. Wertz maintains her previous diagnosis. She is sending Austin to the laboratory at the hospital for a GTT, which has already been scheduled.

Austin's insurance is Blue Cross/Blue Shield. A copy of his card is on file.

Respond to the following questions and perform the listed skills as ordered by Dr. Wertz. *Skills will be accomplished by pairing with a classmate. Role-play the case study where indicated.*

1. Austin is an existing patient and will not require a new patient chart.

2. Identify the diagnosis and all services that must be billed to Austin's insurance company.

   _____

   _____

   _____

   _____

3. Identify the ICD-9-CM (or ICD-10-CM) and CPT codes associated with the items in step 2.

_____

_____

_____

_____

4. Complete an insurance claim form, either manually or using the practice management software, as directed by your instructor. Create the required information such as Austin's address, telephone number, insurance group number, and so on. Your instructor will provide you the fees to use for each item.

5. Submit the completed claim to Dr. Wertz (your instructor) for her signature.

CASE STUDY 65

Patient Education, Injections, Dosage Calculation

© rj lerich/www.Shutterstock.com

Dr. Wertz has diagnosed Austin Garcia with type 1 diabetes; the HbA1c and FBS tests performed at the clinic confirms this diagnosis. (See Case Studies 63 and 64.)

Dr. Wertz would like for you to give Austin an insulin injection. She has also asked you to demonstrate and train Austin and his mother on how to give the injections at home. (Practice with Austin and his mother should be accomplished using sterile saline.)

Dr. Wertz orders Novolog Mix 70/30 100 units/mL 0.5 units/kg daily. Base your dose on Austin weighing 130 lb.

Respond to the following questions and perform the listed skills as ordered by Dr. Wertz. *Skills will be accomplished by pairing with a classmate. Role-play the case study where indicated.*

1. Austin is an existing patient and will not require a new patient chart.

2. Perform medical aseptic hand hygiene and use standard precautions as appropriate.

3. Assemble equipment and supplies.

4. Introduce yourself to the patient.

5. Obtain the proper intake information.

6. Explain the procedure(s).

7. Perform patient assessment including height, weight, TPR, and blood pressure. Use a tympanic thermometer to obtain the patient's temperature.

8. Give Austin the ordered injection. (Research route of injection.)

COMPREHENSIVE

149

9. What special consideration must you take into account before giving Austin the ordered dose of Novolog Mix 70/30?

_____

_____

_____

_____

10. Explain the procedure step by step to Austin (classmate[s]). Demonstrate the procedure and train Austin and his mother on how to give the injections at home. This will include Austin (classmate) giving himself an injection. (Practice with Austin and his mother should be accomplished using sterile saline.)

11. Perform proper hand hygiene. Properly dispose of all waste materials.

12. Record all procedures and results on a SOAP Note form and/or the patient's electronic chart. Submit all documentation to Dr. Wertz (your instructor) for review and evaluation.

CASE STUDY **66**

First Aid–Seizures

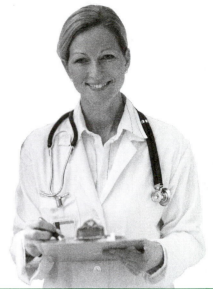

Adam Hutchins arrived at the clinic yesterday, two weeks early, requesting a refill for his muscle relaxants and pain medications. He was referred to a pain clinic and you had a discussion with him about prescription medication abuse and where he might be able to receive help. You documented all information, suspicions, and discussions in his patient record (see Case Study 60).

Adam returns to the clinic today, appearing dysphoric. He is requesting that you "fix him." He is raising his voice and he is blaming you for the pain and discomfort that he is feeling. You explain that Dr. Bledsole is not in the office and that he will need to see another doctor. Adam agrees and says, "Fine. Maybe this doctor will actually do his job! My other doctors don't care if I am in pain!" You notice that Adam has said "other doctors" and make a mental note to write this in his chart, because he only sees Dr. Bledsole at KMC.

You explain to Adam that he will need to sit in the waiting room until an examination room is available. He begins to raise his voice and demands that he be seen right away. Adam is becoming increasingly agitated and begins to vomit in the waiting room. You go to the waiting room and lead Adam back to a sitting area by the examination rooms. As you are leading him, Adam begins to have a seizure.

Chris Taylor, PA, is in the clinic and comes to help. She verifies that there is no Hx of seizures in Adam's record and asks you to call for an ambulance and then obtain an oxygen/nasal cannula, pulse ox, and a nasopharyngeal airway. Chris also requests 5 mg of diazepam (the vial states 5 mg/mL) and IV equipment and supplies (18 gauge catheter, IV tubing, and a bag of LR) as well as a 50 mL bag of D5OW and the blood draw tray.

Respond to the following questions and perform the listed skills. *Skills will be accomplished by pairing with a classmate. Role-play the case study where indicated.*

1. Define dysphoric.

   _____

   _____

   _____

   _____

2. Gather all equipment and supplies required before enacting this scenario. Create a list of the supplies that are necessary for handling this situation. Submit the list to Chris (your instructor).

3. Research and write a one- to two-paragraph paper on the proper way to provide care for a patient during a grand mal seizure.

4. Role-play the case study, beginning with Adam arriving at the clinic today. Include the following:

   - Greeting the patient

   - Explanation of unavailable physician

   - Assisting with a vomiting patient, including clean-up, as needed

   - Medical first aid for grand mal seizures

   - Assessment and triage

   - Vitals

   - Medical asepsis

   - Assisting the physician

   - Calling for an ambulance

5. The seizure has gone on for seven minutes. Chris wants to start the IV, push the diazepam, start the nasopharyngeal airway, and check Adam's blood sugar. (Note: Diazepam cannot be administered until the seizure has occurred for over five minutes.)

6. Hook up and start the oxygen at 4 liters/min. Attach the pulse ox, set up the IV tubing and catheter, draw up the diazepam, and perform a finger stick to assess blood sugar. Adam's blood sugar is 54 mg/dL.

7. Just before Chris starts the IV and administers oxygen Adam vomits again. What should you do?

   _____

   _____

   _____

   _____

8. Chris wants to give the D5OW and to run an ECG. She asks you to prepare the ECG machine.

9. The ambulance arrives before you could perform an ECG. The paramedics take over patient care as Chris updates them on the situation. The paramedics then transport Adam to the hospital for further care.

10. Perform proper hand hygiene. Properly dispose of all waste materials.

11. Address, in writing, everything that has transpired and the medical treatment provided to Adam. Submit it to Chris (your instructor) as a follow-up. Include the following:

    • Patient history

    • Suspicion of substance abuse

    • Initial assessment of patient

    • Treatment as ordered by Chris

12. Document the appropriate information in Adam's chart.

13. Assess emergency preparedness: Did you readily have all equipment and supplies needed. What would you do differently given a similar situation in the future? Discuss in writing and submit it to Chris (your instructor) as a follow-up.

CASE STUDY 67

Patient Termination

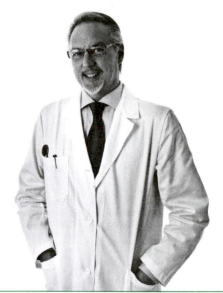

© Minerva Studio/www.Shutterstock.com

Dr. Bledsole has returned to the clinic and you are informing him of the situation concerning Adam Hutchins. You share with Dr. Bledsole that Adam arrived at the clinic a few hours ago suffering from prescription medication withdrawal, during which time Adam made some comments that raised some concerns regarding how he obtained his prescription medications. You explain to Dr. Bledsole that when Adam was informed that he would need to see another doctor his response was, "Fine. Maybe this doctor will actually do his job! My other doctors don't care if I am in pain!" You share your concerns with Dr. Bledsole that he is seeing other doctors for pain medication and provide him with the chart notes you made earlier (in Case Study 66).

Dr. Bledsole agrees with your assessment of the occurrence and would like to terminate Adam as a patient. He would like for you to research for updated guidelines concerning patient termination and then compile them into a report that will act as an official entry in the policy and procedure manual for the clinic. Dr. Bledsole has also requested that you prepare a letter that will serve as notification to Adam of the intent to terminate the physician-patient contract.

Respond to the following questions and perform the listed skills. *Skills will be accomplished by pairing with a classmate. Role-play the case study where indicated.*

1. Role-play the conversation between you and Dr. Bledsole.

2. Research the elements required to withdraw a patient from care.

3. Establish a rough draft of a policy and procedure manual entry for termination of medical care and submit it to Dr. Bledsole (your instructor). Use the watermark function to notate that this is a first draft document. Dr. Bledsole will proofread your document and make suggestions for improvements.

4. When your first draft document is returned, make the required corrections and resubmit your final draft.

5. Prepare the necessary notification and documentation required to terminate the physician-patient contract with Adam for Dr. Bledsole's signature.

6. Dr. Bledsole would like for you to research the quickest and most cost-effective method for mailing the notification of termination to Adam with delivery confirmation via the U.S. Postal Service. Submit your findings to Dr. Bledsole (your instructor).

7. Submit a brief explanation of the various classifications of mail to Dr. Bledsole (your instructor).

8. Prepare the letter to be mailed.

CASE STUDY 68

Job Search–Interview Administration

You are happy with your current position at KMC but would like to explore what other options are out there. There has been no need to update your resume because you have been employed for five years with the clinic. You have not searched for employment and therefore are not up to date on the current search methods. You will also need to freshen up on your interviewing skills.

Respond to the following questions and perform the listed skills. *Skills will be accomplished by pairing with a classmate. Role-play the case study where indicated.*

1. Create or update your current resume. Submit a first draft to your instructor.

2. Perform a job search. (These positions must be different than the positions located in a previous case study.)

   a. Locate a minimum of two positions you are qualified for in the local paper.

   b. Locate a minimum of two positions you are qualified for using the Internet.

   c. Locate a minimum of two positions you are qualified for using networking.

   d. Submit documentation of positions to your instructor.

3. Write an appropriate cover letter for the position you located above that you are most interested in interviewing for.

4. Request an interview by telephone by role-playing with a classmate.

5. Interview. (Your instructor will arrange for interviews with a school administrator or other instructor to accomplish the interview portion of this case study.)

6. Follow-up with a thank-you card. Submit it to the school administrator who interviewed you. Submit a copy also to your instructor.

CASE STUDY 69

Annual Evaluation

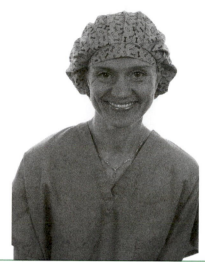

It is time for yearly evaluations. Dr. Wertz will be conducting the evaluations this year. However, all of the physicians will review your self-evaluation form and submit their input on your performance for the past year. This is a two-part process. First, you are required to complete the self-evaluation form provided to you by Dr. Wertz (your instructor). Second, Dr. Wertz will conduct a personal interview, where the two of you will evaluate your performance, review your self-evaluation, and discuss comments from the other practitioners for the past year.

Respond to the following questions and perform the listed skills. *Skills will be accomplished by interviewing with Dr. Wertz (your instructor). Role-play the case study where indicated.*

1. Complete the self-evaluation form provided by your instructor in the given time frame. Answer the questions based on your performance as a medical assistant during the completion of the assigned case studies. Your instructor will then review your evaluation as if you were an actual medical assistant employee, provide feedback, and schedule a time for your interview.

2. Schedule and attend your evaluation interview.

CASE STUDY **SUPPLEMENT**

Insurance Billing and Coding

The following can be used as a supplement to many of the case studies when additional insurance billing and coding practice is desired. Your instructor will assign this supplement where he or she deems appropriate.

Your instructor will determine the insurance carrier for the case study and provide you with the billing information.

Read through the case study's content and apply it to the following questions.

Respond to the following questions and perform the listed skills as ordered by the case study's health care practitioner. *Skills will be accomplished by pairing with a classmate. Role-play the case study where indicated.*

1. Identify if the patient is a new patient or an existing patient. If a new patient, the patient chart will be created as part of the initial case study.

2. Identify the diagnosis and all services that must be billed to the patient's insurance company.

3. Identify the ICD-9-CM or ICD-10-CM and CPT codes associated with the patient's diagnosis and each of the services.

4. Complete an insurance claim form, either manually or using practice management software, as directed by your instructor. Create the required information such as the patient's address, telephone number, insurance group number, and so on. Your instructor will provide you the fees to use for each item.

5. Submit the completed claim to the health care practitioner associated with the case study (your instructor) for his or her signature.

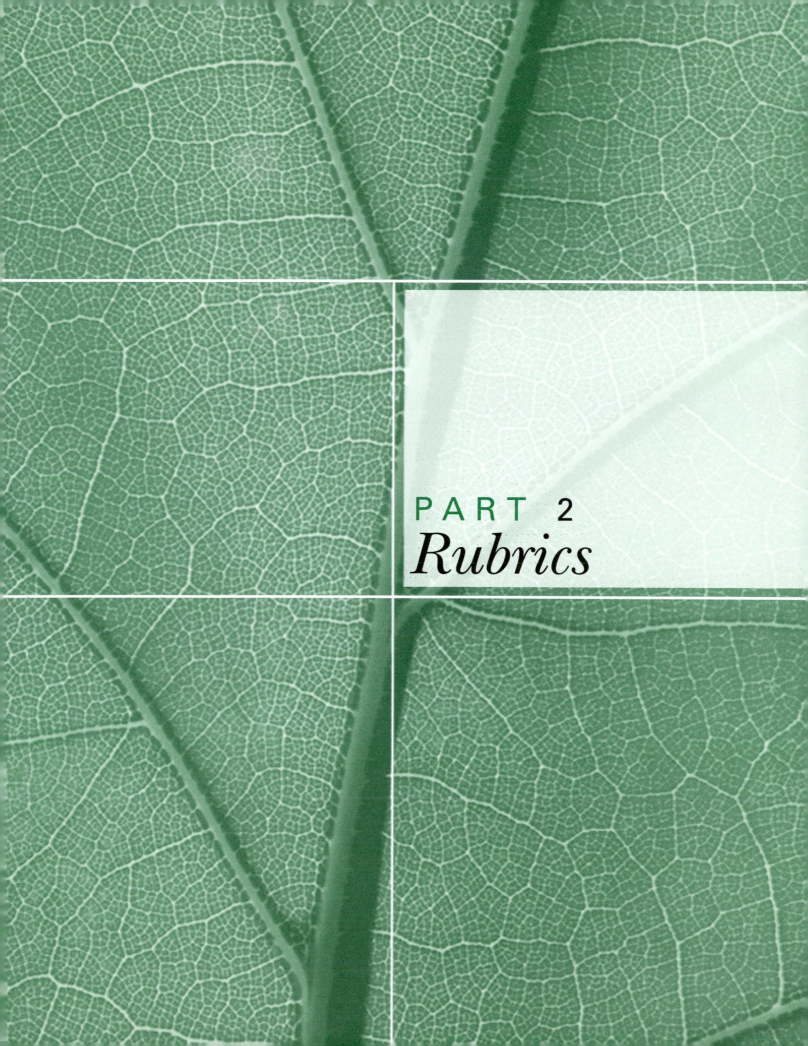

PART 2
Rubrics

Medical Assistant Responsibilities

Name _____ Date _____

Elements	4 Excellent	3 Proficient	2 Adequate	1 Needs Improvement	Points
General List of Responsibilities Divided by Administrative and Clinical Duties	Student responded appropriately to step 1 with one or less errors.	Student responded appropriately to step 1 with two errors.	Student responded appropriately to step 1 with three to four errors.	Student failed to respond appropriately to step 1 or did so with five or more errors.	
Assign Responsibilities	Student responded appropriately to step 2 with one or less errors.	Student responded appropriately to step 2 with two errors.	Student responded appropriately to step 2 with three to four errors.	Student failed to respond appropriately to step 2 or did so with five or more errors.	
Prioritization of Responsibilities	Student responded appropriately to step 3 with one or less errors.	Student responded appropriately to step 3 with two errors.	Student responded appropriately to step 3 with three to four errors.	Student failed to respond appropriately to step 3 or did so with five or more errors.	
Final Draft of Written Document of Responsibilities	Student responded appropriately to step 4 with one or less errors.	Student responded appropriately to step 4 with two errors.	Student responded appropriately to step 4 with three to four errors.	Student failed to respond appropriately to step 4 or did so with five or more errors.	
Appointment Schedule	Student appropriately created appointments for 11 patients with one or less errors.	Student appropriately created appointments for 11 patients with two errors.	Student appropriately created appointments for 11 patients with three to four errors.	Student failed to appropriately create appointments for 11 patients or did so with five or more errors.	
Preparation of Reception Area and Examination Rooms	Student appropriately prepared the reception area and two examination rooms, either physically or in writing, with one or less errors.	Student appropriately prepared the reception area and two examination rooms, either physically or in writing, with two errors.	Student appropriately prepared the reception area and two examination rooms, either physically or in writing, with three to four errors.	Student failed to appropriately prepare the reception area and two examination rooms, either physically or in writing, or did so with five or more errors.	
Overtime Arrangements	Student appropriately provided a written document describing what accommodations he or she would personally need to make to work three hours of overtime.	N/A	N/A	Student failed to appropriately provide a written document describing what accommodations he or she would personally need to make to work three hours of overtime.	

Description of Conflict	Student appropriately provided a written document describing any conflict that occurred during this case study either through role-play or in actuality, or if no conflict occurred, and this is acknowledged, a description of the conflict that may have occurred given a different partner or future coworker.	N/A	N/A	Student failed to appropriately provide a written document describing any conflict that occurred during this case study either through role-play or in actuality, or if no conflict occurred, and this is acknowledged, a description of the conflict that may have occurred given a different partner or future coworker.
				TOTAL

Based on the above criteria the student's grade for this assignment is: _____

(Total the points for each element scored and average for a final grade.)

Comments to the Student:

Instructor Signature: _____   Date: _____

Administrative Duties and Telephone Techniques–Day 1

Name _____

Date _____

Elements	4 Excellent	3 Proficient	2 Adequate	1 Needs Improvement	Points
Telephone Greeting and Introduction of Office and Self	Student appropriately greeted and introduced the office and self to the patient with one or less errors.	Student appropriately greeted and introduced the office and self to the patient with two errors.	Student appropriately greeted and introduced the office and self to the patient with three to four errors.	Student failed to appropriately greet and introduce the office and self to the patient or did so with five or more errors.	
Demonstrating Multiple-Line Competency	Student demonstrated competency in this skill with one or less errors.	Student demonstrated competency in this skill with two errors.	Student demonstrated competency in this skill with three to four errors.	Student failed to demonstrate this competency or did so with five or more errors.	
Telephone Call Screening	Student accurately screened all five telephone calls.	Student accurately screened four telephone calls.	Student accurately screened three telephone calls.	Student accurately screened one to two telephone calls or failed to screen any telephone calls.	
Gathering Data over the Telephone with Patient Interview/ Questioning Techniques	Student gathered pertinent patient data while using interview questioning techniques with no errors.	Student gathered pertinent patient data while using interview questioning techniques with one to two errors.	Student gathered pertinent patient data while using interview questioning techniques with three to four errors.	Student gathered pertinent patient data while using interview questioning techniques with five or more errors or failed to gather pertinent information from the patient.	
Evaluating the Effectiveness of Patient Interviewing Techniques	Student employed observational and active listening skills and provided appropriate feedback with one or less errors.	Student employed observational and active listening skills and provided appropriate feedback with two errors.	Student employed observational and active listening skills and provided appropriate feedback with three to four errors.	Student employed observational and active listening skills and provided appropriate feedback with five or more errors.	
Obtaining and Documenting Telephone Messages	Student properly documented all information obtained with one or less errors.	Student documented all information obtained with two errors.	Student documented all information obtained with three errors.	Student documented all information obtained with four or more errors or failed to obtain and document information.	

Appointment Scheduling	Student correctly scheduled an appointment and obtained the required information with one or less errors.	Students correctly scheduled an appointment and obtained the required information with two errors.	Student correctly scheduled an appointment and obtained the required information with three to four errors.	Student failed to correctly schedule an appointment and/or failed to obtain the required information or did so with five or more errors.
Ending Telephone Calls	Student professionally ended all telephone calls with one or less errors.	Student professionally ended all telephone calls with two errors.	Student professionally ended all telephone calls with three errors.	Student professionally ended all telephone calls with four or more errors or failed to professionally end any telephone calls.
				TOTAL

Based on the above criteria the student's grade for this assignment is: _____

(Total the points for each element scored and average for a final grade.)

Comments to the Student:

Instructor Signature: _____   Date: _____

CASE STUDY **3**   *Administrative Duties and Telephone Techniques–Day 2*

Name _____   Date _____

Elements	4 Excellent	3 Proficient	2 Adequate	1 Needs Improvement	Points
Telephone Greeting and Introduction of Office and Self	Student appropriately greeted and introduced the office and self to the patient with one or less errors.	Student appropriately greeted and introduced the office and self to the patient with two errors.	Student appropriately greeted and introduced the office and self to the patient with three to four errors.	Student failed to appropriately greet and introduce the office and self to the patient or did so with five or more errors.	
Transferring Calls	Student demonstrated competency in transferring calls.	N/A	N/A	Student failed to demonstrate competency in transferring calls.	
Telephone Call Screening	Student effectively gathered information while screening with no errors.	Student effectively gathered information while screening with one error.	Student effectively gathered information while screening with two errors.	Student effectively gathered information while screening with three or more errors or failed to perform this task.	
Scenario 1 Patient Confidentiality and Professionalism	Student demonstrated competency in maintaining patient confidentiality and professionalism.	N/A	N/A	Student failed to demonstrate competency in maintaining patient confidentiality and professionalism.	
Schedule and Provide Patient with Follow-up Appointment Time	Student appropriately performed these tasks with one or less errors.	Student appropriately performed these tasks with two errors.	Student appropriately performed these tasks with three errors.	Student failed to appropriately perform these tasks or did so with four or more errors.	
Scenario 1 Research Report	Student researched and developed a quality one-page report with one or less errors.	Student researched and developed a quality one-page report with two errors.	Student researched and developed a quality one-page report with three to four errors.	Student researched and developed a quality one-page report with five or more errors or failed to complete this task.	
Reminder Call and Telephone Techniques	Student correctly completed a reminder call with proper techniques with one or less errors.	Student correctly completed a reminder call with proper techniques with no more than two errors.	Student correctly completed a reminder call with proper techniques with no more than three to four errors.	Student failed to correctly complete a reminder call with proper techniques or did so with five or more errors.	
Scenario 2 Patient Confidentiality and Professionalism	Student demonstrated competency in maintaining patient confidentiality and professionalism.	N/A	N/A	Student failed to demonstrate competency in maintaining patient confidentiality and professionalism.	

Criteria					Points
Professional Communication with a Patient Who Is Elderly and Hard of Hearing	Student demonstrated the ability to professionally communicate with a patient who is elderly and hard of hearing with one or less errors.	Student demonstrated the ability to professionally communicate with a patient who is elderly and hard of hearing with two errors.	Student demonstrated the ability to professionally communicate with a patient who is elderly and hard of hearing with three to four errors.	Student demonstrated the ability to professionally communicate with a patient who is elderly and hard of hearing with five or more errors or failed to professionally communicate with a patient who is elderly and hard of hearing.	
Scenario 2 Research Report	Student researched and developed a quality one-page report with one or less errors.	Student researched and developed a quality one-page report with two errors.	Student researched and developed a quality one-page report with three to four errors.	Student researched and developed a quality one-page report with five or more errors or failed to complete this task.	
Appointment Scheduling	Student correctly scheduled an appointment and obtained the required information with one or less errors.	Students correctly scheduled an appointment and obtained the required information with two errors.	Student correctly scheduled an appointment and obtained the required information with three to four errors.	Student failed to correctly schedule an appointment and/or failed to obtain the required information or did so with five or more errors.	
					TOTAL

Based on the above criteria the student's grade for this assignment is: _____

(Total the points for each element scored and average for a final grade.)

Comments to the Student:

Instructor Signature: _____ Date: _____

Body Divisions, Planes, Positions, Draping/Gowning, and Ethics

Name _____ Date _____

Elements	4 Excellent	3 Proficient	2 Adequate	1 Needs Improvement	Points
Fundamental Writing Skills	Student submitted a written document with one or less errors.	Student submitted a written document with two errors.	Student submitted a written document with three errors.	Student failed to submit a written document or did so with four or more errors.	
Terminology	Student correctly selected, spelled, and used the appropriate terminology for the assignment with no errors.	Student correctly selected, spelled, and used the appropriate terminology for the assignment with one error.	Student correctly selected, spelled, and used the appropriate terminology for the assignment with two errors.	Student failed to correctly select, spell, or use the appropriate terminology for the assignment or did so with three or more errors.	
Reference Sources	Student correctly referenced sources with no errors.	Student correctly referenced sources with one error.	Student correctly referenced sources with two errors.	Student failed to correctly reference sources or did so with three or more errors.	
Researched Presentation	Student correctly presented the required information with no errors.	Student correctly presented the required information with one error.	Student correctly presented the required information with two errors.	Student failed to correctly present the required information or did so with three or more errors.	
Visual Presentation	Student prepared a visual presentation with no errors.	Student prepared a visual presentation with one error.	Student prepared a visual presentation with two errors.	Student failed to present a visual presentation or did so with three or more errors.	
Professional Communication	Student properly addressed professional communication with patients with no errors.	Student properly addressed professional communication with patients with one error.	Student properly addressed professional communication with patients with two errors.	Student failed to properly address professional communication with patients or did so with three or more errors.	
Ethics	Student appropriately presented ethical standards when addressing patients with no errors.	Student appropriately presented ethical standards when addressing patients with one error.	Student appropriately presented ethical standards with addressing patients with two errors.	Student failed to appropriately present ethical standards or did so with three or more errors.	
Criminal/Unprofessional Conduct and Liability	Student correctly addressed criminal/unprofessional conduct and liability with one or less errors.	Student correctly addressed criminal/unprofessional conduct and liability with two errors.	Student correctly addressed criminal/unprofessional conduct and liability with three errors.	Student failed to correctly address criminal/unprofessional conduct and liability or did so with four or more errors.	

	Student applied professional communication skills during oral presentation with no errors.	Student applied professional communication skills during oral presentation with one error.	Student applied professional communication skills during oral presentation with two errors.	Student failed to apply professional communication skills or did so with three or more errors.	
Oral Presentation					
Policy and Procedures Manual Written Submission	Student submitted a document to be entered into the policy and procedures manual with no errors.	Student submitted a document to be entered into the policy and procedures manual with one error.	Student submitted a document to be entered into the policy and procedures manual with two errors.	Student failed to submit a document to be entered into the policy and procedures manual or did so with three or more errors.	
				TOTAL	

Based on the above criteria the student's grade for this assignment is: _____

(Total the points for each element scored and average for a final grade.)

Comments to the Student:

Instructor Signature: _____ Date: _____

Filing—Medical Records

Name _____ Date _____

Elements	4 Excellent	3 Proficient	2 Adequate	1 Needs Improvement	Points
Explain and Demonstrate Basic Filing Systems	Student correctly explained and demonstrated basic filing systems with one or less errors.	Student correctly explained and demonstrated basic filing systems with two errors.	Student correctly explained and demonstrated basic filing systems with three errors.	Student failed to correctly explain and demonstrate basic filing systems or did so with four or more errors.	
Explain and Demonstrate Special Filing Systems	Student correctly explained and demonstrated special filing systems with one or less errors.	Student correctly explained and demonstrated special filing systems with two errors.	Student correctly explained and demonstrated special filing systems with three errors.	Student failed to correctly explain and demonstrate special filing systems or did so with four or more errors.	
Explain and Demonstrate Filing Guidelines	Student correctly explained and demonstrated filing guidelines with one or less errors.	Student correctly explained and demonstrated filing guidelines with two errors.	Student correctly explained and demonstrated filing guidelines with three errors.	Student failed to explain and demonstrate filing guidelines or did so with four or more errors.	
Explain and Demonstrate Medical Record Organization	Student correctly explained and demonstrated medical record organization with one or less errors.	Student correctly explained and demonstrated medical record organization with two errors.	Student correctly explained and demonstrated medical record organization with three errors.	Student failed to correctly explain and demonstrate medical record organization or did so with four or more errors.	
Explain the Types of Medical Records	Student correctly explained the types of medical records with no errors.	Student correctly explained the types of medical records with one error.	Student correctly explained the types of medical records with two errors.	Student failed to correctly explain the type of medical records or did so with three or more errors.	
Explain and Demonstrate Collecting Information for Medical Records	Student correctly explained and demonstrated collecting information for medical records with one or less errors.	Student correctly explained and demonstrated collecting information for medical records with two errors.	Student correctly explained and demonstrated collecting information for medical records with three errors.	Student failed to correctly explain or demonstrate collecting information for medical records or did so with four or more errors.	

Explain and Demonstrate Making Medical Record Corrections	Student correctly explained and demonstrated making medical record corrections with no errors.	Student correctly explained and demonstrated making medical record corrections with one error.	Student correctly explained and demonstrated making medical record corrections with two errors.	Student failed to correctly explain and demonstrate making medical record corrections or did so with three or more errors.
Explain the Retaining and Purging of Medical Records	Student correctly explained the retaining and purging of medical records with one or less errors.	Student correctly explained the retaining and purging of medical records with two errors.	Student correctly explained the retaining and purging of medical records with three errors.	Student failed to correctly explain the retaining and purging of medical records or did so with four or more errors.
				TOTAL

Based on the above criteria the student's grade for this assignment is: _____

(Total the points for each element scored and average for a final grade.)

Comments to the Student:

Instructor Signature: _____   Date: _____

CASE STUDY 6   *Equipment Supply and Inventory*

Name _____ Date _____

Elements	4 Excellent	3 Proficient	2 Adequate	1 Needs Improvement	Points
Inventory of Clinical Supplies and Equipment	Student completed the inventory with no errors.	Student completed the inventory with one error.	Student completed the inventory with two errors.	Student failed to complete the inventory or did so with three or more errors.	
Research of Vendors	Student located and researched two clinical product vendors.	N/A	N/A	Student failed to locate and research vendors or only located and researched one vendor.	
Itemized List of Cost of Supplies and Equipment	Student located and researched the cost of the listed products and produced an itemized list with no errors.	Student located and researched the cost of the listed products and produced an itemized list with two errors.	Student located and researched the cost of the listed products and produced an itemized list with three or four errors.	Student failed to locate and research the cost of the listed products and produce an itemized list or did so with five or more errors.	
Faxed Purchase Order	Student demonstrated correct usage of the fax machine with no errors.	Student demonstrated correct usage of the fax machine with one error.	Student demonstrated correct usage of the fax machine with two errors.	Student failed to demonstrate correct usage of the fax machine or did so with three or more errors.	
				TOTAL	

Based on the above criteria the student's grade for this assignment is: _____

(Total the points for each element scored and average for a final grade.)

Comments to the Student:

Instructor Signature: _____ Date: _____

CASE STUDY 7 *Administrative Duties and Training*

Name _____ Date _____

Elements	4 Excellent	3 Proficient	2 Adequate	1 Needs Improvement	Points
Explain and Demonstrate Protocols for Answering the Telephone	Student correctly explained and demonstrated protocols for answering the telephone with one or less errors.	Student correctly explained and demonstrated protocols for answering the telephone with two errors.	Student correctly explained and demonstrated protocols for answering the telephone with three errors.	Student explained and demonstrated protocols for answering the telephone with four or more errors.	
Explain and Demonstrate Protocols for Taking Messages	Student correctly explained and demonstrated protocols for taking messages with one or less errors.	Student correctly explained and demonstrated protocols for taking messages with two errors.	Student correctly explained and demonstrated protocols for taking messages with three errors.	Student correctly explained and demonstrated protocols for taking messages with four or more errors.	
Explain and Demonstrate Protocols for Confirming Appointments	Student correctly explained and demonstrated protocols for confirming appointments with one or less errors.	Student correctly explained and demonstrated protocols for confirming appointments with two errors.	Student correctly explained and demonstrated protocols for confirming appointments with three errors.	Student correctly explained and demonstrated protocols for confirming appointments with four or more errors.	
Explain and Demonstrate Scheduling Appointments	Student correctly explained and demonstrated protocols for scheduling appointments with one or less errors.	Student correctly explained and demonstrated protocols for scheduling appointments with two errors.	Student correctly explained and demonstrated protocols for scheduling appointments with three errors.	Student correctly explained and demonstrated protocols for scheduling appointments with four or more errors.	
Explain and Demonstrate How to Matrix the Appointment Book	Student correctly explained and demonstrated how to matrix the appointment book with no errors.	Student correctly explained and demonstrated how to matrix the appointment book with one error.	Student correctly explained and demonstrated how to matrix the appointment book with two errors.	Student correctly explained and demonstrated how to matrix the appointment book with three or more errors.	
Observe and Provide Constructive Criticism	Student displayed professionalism while observing and providing relevant constructive criticism.	N/A	N/A	Student failed to display professionalism while observing and providing relevant constructive criticism or displayed professionalism while observing but failed to provide relevant constructive criticism or displayed professionalism while providing constructive criticism but failed to display professionalism while observing.	
				TOTAL	

Based on the above criteria the student's grade for this assignment is: _____

(Total the points for each element scored and average for a final grade.)

Comments to the Student:

Instructor Signature: _____ Date: _____

CASE STUDY 8 *Processing Incoming Mail and Posting Payments*

Name _____ Date _____

Elements	4 Excellent	3 Proficient	2 Adequate	1 Needs Improvement	Points
Prioritize Incoming Mail	Student correctly prioritized incoming mail with no errors.	Student correctly prioritized incoming mail with one error.	Student correctly prioritized incoming mail with two errors.	Student failed to correctly prioritize incoming mail or did so with three or more errors.	
Processing Mail	Student correctly explained how each piece of mail should be processed and dispatched with one or less errors.	Student correctly explained how each piece of mail should be processed and dispatched with two errors.	Student correctly explained how each piece of mail should be processed and dispatched with three errors.	Student failed to correctly explain how each piece of mail should be processed and dispatched or did so with four or more errors.	
Posting Collection Agency Data	Student correctly posted collection agency data to patient accounts with no errors.	Student correctly posted collection agency data to patient accounts with one error.	Student correctly posted collection agency data to patient accounts with two errors.	Student failed to correctly post collection agency data to patient accounts or did so with three or more errors.	
Posting Payments to Patient Accounts	Student correctly posted payments to patient accounts with one or less errors.	Student correctly posted payments to patient accounts with two errors.	Student correctly posted payments to patient accounts with three errors.	Student failed to correctly post payments to patient accounts or did so with four or more errors.	
				TOTAL	

Based on the above criteria the student's grade for this assignment is: _____
(Total the points for each element scored and average for a final grade.)

Comments to the Student:

Instructor Signature: _____ Date: _____

Research for Presentation

Name _____ Date _____

Elements	4 Excellent	3 Proficient	2 Adequate	1 Needs Improvement	Points
Internet Search	Student correctly performed an Internet search and located at least two reports or studies conducted by physicians dated within the past 12 months with one or less errors.	Student correctly performed an Internet search and located at least two reports or studies conducted by physicians dated within the past 12 months with two errors.	Student correctly performed an Internet search and located at least two reports or studies conducted by physicians dated within the past 12 months with three to four errors.	Student failed to correctly perform an Internet search or did not locate at least two reports or studies conducted by physicians dated within the past 12 months or did so with five or more errors.	
Physician Contact Information	Student appropriately located three sources of contact information for physician(s) authoring reports or studies.	Student appropriately located two sources of contact information for physician(s) authoring reports or studies.	Student appropriately located one source of contact information for physician(s) authoring reports or studies.	Student failed to appropriately locate contact information for physician(s) authoring reports or studies.	
Report–First Draft	Student appropriately submitted a first draft of a 500-word report taking a stand either supporting or denying the effectiveness of the use of antioxidants in treating prostate cancer with one or less errors.	Student appropriately submitted a first draft of a 500-word report taking a stand either supporting or denying the effectiveness of the use of antioxidants in treating prostate cancer with two errors.	Student appropriately submitted a first draft of a 500-word report taking a stand either supporting or denying the effectiveness of the use of antioxidants in treating prostate cancer with three to four errors.	Student failed to appropriately submit a first draft of a 500-word report taking a stand either supporting or denying the effectiveness of the use of antioxidants in treating prostate cancer or did so with five or more errors.	
Report–First Draft	Student appropriately used the MLA or APA format for report writing and correctly cited the source articles supporting his or her view with one or less errors.	Student appropriately used the MLA or APA format for report writing and correctly cited the source articles supporting his or her view with two errors.	Student appropriately used the MLA or APA format for report writing and correctly cited the source articles supporting his or her view with three to four errors.	Student failed to appropriately use the MLA or APA format for report writing and correctly cite the source articles supporting his or her view or did so with five or more errors.	
Report–First Draft	Student appropriately used medical terminology, sentence structure, grammar, and punctuation with one to two errors.	Student appropriately used medical terminology, sentence structure, grammar, and punctuation with two to three errors.	Student appropriately used medical terminology, sentence structure, grammar, and punctuation with four to five errors.	Student failed to appropriately use medical terminology, sentence structure, grammar, and punctuation or did so with five or more errors.	
Report–Final Draft	Student appropriately corrected the first draft based on the instructor's feedback and resubmitted the report with one to two errors.	Student appropriately corrected the first draft based on the instructor's feedback and resubmitted the report with two to three errors.	Student appropriately corrected the first draft based on the instructor's feedback and resubmitted the report with four to five errors.	Student failed to appropriately correct the first draft based on the instructor's feedback and resubmit the report or did so with five or more errors.	
				TOTAL	

Based on the above criteria the student's grade for this assignment is: _____

(Total the points for each element scored and average for a final grade.)

Comments to the Student:

Instructor Signature: _____ Date: _____

CASE STUDY 10 *Banking Procedures and Preparing Outgoing Mail*

Name _____ Date _____

Elements	4 Excellent	3 Proficient	2 Adequate	1 Needs Improvement	Points
Prepare Checks for Payments Due	Student correctly prepared the checks for the payments due with one or less errors.	Student correctly prepared the checks for the payments due with two errors.	Student correctly prepared the checks for the payments due with three errors.	Student failed to correctly prepare the checks for the payments due or did so with four or more errors.	
Outgoing Mail	Student correctly prepared the payments due for outgoing mail with one or less errors.	Student correctly prepared the payments due for outgoing mail with two errors.	Student correctly prepared the payments due for outgoing mail with three errors.	Student failed to correctly prepare the payments due for outgoing mail or did so with four or more errors.	
Prepare Bank Deposit	Student correctly prepared the bank deposit with no errors.	Student correctly prepared the bank deposit with one error.	Student correctly prepared the bank deposit with two errors.	Student failed to correctly prepare the bank deposit or did so with three or more errors.	
Reconcile Bank Statement	Student correctly reconciled the bank statement with one or less errors.	Student correctly reconciled the bank statement with two errors.	Student correctly reconciled the bank statement with three errors.	Student failed to correctly reconcile the bank statement or did so with four or more errors.	
				TOTAL	

Based on the above criteria the student's grade for this assignment is: _____
(Total the points for each element scored and average for a final grade.)

Comments to the Student:

Instructor Signature: _____   Date: _____

Follow-Up Appointments

Name _____ Date _____

Elements	4 Excellent	3 Proficient	2 Adequate	1 Needs Improvement	Points
Reminder Call and Telephone Techniques	Student correctly completed a reminder call with proper techniques with one or less errors.	Student correctly completed a reminder call with proper techniques with no more than two errors.	Student correctly completed a reminder call with proper techniques with no more than three to four errors.	Student failed to correctly complete a reminder call with proper techniques or did so with five or more errors.	
Research and Development of Questions	Student researched and developed 10 questions.	Student researched and developed eight to nine questions.	Student researched and developed six to seven questions.	Students researched and developed five questions or failed to research and develop any questions.	
Quality and Types of Questions	Student developed quality exploratory, open-ended, and direct questions.	Student developed quality questions but only used two of the three types of questions.	Student developed quality questions but only used one of the three types of questions.	Student failed to develop quality questions of any type.	
Introduction to Patient	Student appropriately introduced self to the patient with one or less errors.	Student appropriately introduced self to the patient with two errors.	Student appropriately introduced self to the patient with three to four errors.	Student failed to appropriately introduce self to the patient or did so with five or more errors.	
Evaluating the Effectiveness of Patient Interviewing Techniques	Student employed observational and active listening skills and provided appropriate feedback with one or less errors.	Student employed observational and active listening skills and provided appropriate feedback with two errors.	Student employed observational and active listening skills and provided appropriate feedback with three to four errors.	Student employed observational and active listening skills and provided appropriate feedback with five or more errors.	
Documentation	Student properly documented all information obtained with one or less errors.	Student properly documented all information obtained with two errors or omitted documentation of one to two answered questions.	Student properly documented all information obtained with three to four errors or omitted documentation of two answered questions.	Student properly documented all information obtained with five or more errors or omitted documentation of three or more answered questions.	
Schedule and Provide Patient with Follow-up Appointment Time	Student appropriately performed these tasks with one or less errors.	Student appropriately performed these tasks with two errors.	Student appropriately performed these tasks with three errors.	Student failed to appropriately perform these tasks or did so with four or more errors.	
				TOTAL	

Based on the above criteria the student's grade for this assignment is: _____

(Total the points for each element scored and average for a final grade.)

Comments to the Student:

Instructor Signature: _____ Date: _____

CASE STUDY 12   *Community Outreach Interview*

Name _____   Date _____

Elements	4 Excellent	3 Proficient	2 Adequate	1 Needs Improvement	Points
Role-Play Scenario 1	Student participated in the role-play.	N/A	N/A	Student failed to participate in the role-play.	
Microbiology and Its Impact	Student accurately defined microbiology and explained its impact within a health care facility with no errors.	Student accurately defined microbiology and explained its impact within a health care facility with one error.	Student accurately defined microbiology and explained its impact within a health care facility with two errors.	Student failed to accurately define microbiology and explain its impact within a health care facility or did so with three or more errors.	
Pathogens	Student correctly identified and described the five main pathogens with no errors.	Student correctly identified and described the five main pathogens with one error.	Student correctly identified and described the five main pathogens with two errors.	Student failed to correctly identify and describe the five main pathogens or did so with three or more errors.	
Pathogens and the Disease Process	Student provided an example of each pathogen as it pertains to the disease process within the clinic with no errors.	Student provided an example of each pathogen as it pertains to the disease process within the clinic with one error.	Student provided an example of each pathogen as it pertains to the disease process within the clinic with two errors.	Student failed to provide an example of each pathogen as it pertains to the disease process within the clinic or did so with three or more errors.	
Gram Staining	Student appropriately responded to the questions regarding Gram staining with one or less errors.	Student appropriately responded to the questions regarding Gram staining with two errors.	Student appropriately responded to the questions regarding Gram staining with three errors.	Student failed to appropriately respond to the questions regarding Gram staining or did so with four or more errors.	
Overview of Interview Questions	Student submitted an overview of his or her responses to the interview questions.	N/A	N/A	Student failed to submit an overview of his or her responses to the interview questions.	
				TOTAL	

Based on the above criteria the student's grade for this assignment is: _____

(Total the points for each element scored and average for a final grade.)

Comments to the Student:

Instructor Signature: _____ Date: _____

Ordering Administrative Equipment and Supplies

Name _____ Date _____

Elements	4 Excellent	3 Proficient	2 Adequate	1 Needs Improvement	Points
Inventory of Administrative Supplies and Equipment	Student completed the inventory with no errors.	Student completed the inventory with one error.	Student completed the inventory with two errors.	Student failed to complete the inventory or did so with three or more errors.	
Research of Vendors	Student located and researched two clinical product vendors.	N/A	N/A	Student failed to locate and research vendors or only located and researched one vendor.	
Itemized List of Cost of Supplies and Equipment	Student located and researched the cost of the listed products and produced an itemized list with no errors.	Student located and researched the cost of the listed products and produced an itemized list with two errors.	Student located and researched the cost of the listed products and produced and itemized list with three to four errors.	Student failed to locate and research the cost of the listed products or did so with five or more errors.	
Telephone Purchase Order	Student demonstrated the ability to place an order via the telephone with no errors.	Student demonstrated the ability to place an order via the telephone with one error.	Student demonstrated the ability to place an order via the telephone with two errors.	Student failed to demonstrate the ability to place an order via the telephone or did so with three or more errors.	
				TOTAL	

Based on the above criteria the student's grade for this assignment is: _____

(Total the points for each element scored and average for a final grade.)

Comments to the Student:

Instructor Signature: _____ Date: _____

Consent for Release of Medical Records

Name _____ Date _____

Elements	4 Excellent	3 Proficient	2 Adequate	1 Needs Improvement	Points
Role-Play Question 1	Student participated in the role-play scenario.	N/A	N/A	Student failed to participate in the role-play scenario.	
Telephone Greeting and Introduction of Office and Self	Student appropriately greeted and introduced the office and self with no errors.	N/A	N/A	Student failed to appropriately greet and introduce the office and self.	
Explanation for Consent	Student explained the need for consent with no errors.	Student explained the need for consent with one error.	Student explained the need for consent with two errors.	Student failed to explain the need for consent or did so with three or more errors.	
Maintaining Confidentiality	Student maintained patient confidentiality while role-playing the telephone conversation.	N/A	N/A	Student failed to maintain patient confidentiality while role-playing the telephone conversation.	
Ending Telephone Call	Student professionally ended the telephone call with no errors.	N/A	N/A	Student failed to professionally end the telephone call or did so with errors.	
Response to Question 2	Student responded appropriately to question 2 with one or less errors.	Student responded appropriately to question 2 with two errors.	Student responded appropriately to question 2 with three errors.	Student failed to respond appropriately to question 2 or did so with four or more errors.	
Role-Play Question 3	Student participated in the role-play scenario.	N/A	N/A	Student failed to participate in the role-play scenario.	
Telephone Greeting and Introduction of Office and Self	Student appropriately greeted and introduced the office and self with no errors.	N/A	N/A	Student failed to appropriately greet and introduce the office and self.	
Maintaining Confidentiality	Student maintained patient confidentiality while role-playing the telephone conversation.	N/A	N/A	Student failed to maintain patient confidentiality while role-playing the telephone conversation.	
Ending Telephone Call	Student professionally ended the telephone call with no errors.	N/A	N/A	Student failed to professionally end the telephone call or did so with errors.	
Consent Form	Student accurately completed a consent form for the release of patient medical records with one or less errors.	Student accurately completed a consent form for the release of patient medical records with two errors.	Student accurately completed a consent form for the release of patient medical records with three errors.	Student failed to accurately complete a consent form for the release of patient medical records or did so with four or more errors.	

Fax Machine	Student demonstrated the ability to fax the consent form with no errors.	N/A	N/A	Student failed to demonstrate the ability to fax the consent form.	
Copy Patient Records	Student copied the correct portion of the patient's medical record with one or less errors.	Student copied the correct portion of the patient's medical record with two errors.	Student copied the correct portion of the patient's medical record with three to four errors.	Student failed to copy the correct portion of the patient's medical record or did so with five or more errors.	
Prepare Records for Overnight Delivery	Student accurately prepared the patient's medical record for overnight delivery.	N/A	N/A	Student failed to accurately prepare the patient's medical record for overnight delivery.	
				TOTAL	

Based on the above criteria the student's grade for this assignment is: _____

(Total the points for each element scored and average for a final grade.)

Comments to the Student:

Instructor Signature: _____   Date: _____

Communication with a Distraught Patient

Name _____

Date _____

Elements	4 Excellent	3 Proficient	2 Adequate	1 Needs Improvement	Points
Telephone Greeting and Introduction of Office and Self	Student appropriately greeted and introduced the office and self to the patient with one or less errors.	Student appropriately greeted and introduced the office and self to the patient with two errors.	Student appropriately greeted and introduced the office and self to the patient with three to four errors.	Student failed to appropriately greet and introduce the office and self to the patient or did so with five or more errors.	
Communication with Distraught Patient	Student demonstrated the ability to professionally communicate with a distraught patient.	N/A	N/A	Student failed to demonstrate the ability to professionally communicate with a distraught patient.	
Evaluating for Effectiveness	Student employed observational and active listening skills and provided appropriate feedback with one or less errors.	Student employed observational and active listening skills and provided appropriate feedback with two errors.	Student employed observational and active listening skills and provided appropriate feedback with three to four errors.	Student failed to employ observational and active listening skills and provide appropriate feedback or did so with five or more errors.	
Writing Assignment in Step 2	Student submitted the required information in a grammatically correct paper with at least three paragraphs.	Student submitted the required information with grammatical errors in a paper with three paragraphs or submitted the required information in a grammatically correct paper with at least two paragraphs.	Student submitted the required information with grammatical errors in a paper with two paragraphs or submitted the required information in a grammatically correct paper with at least one paragraph.	Student failed to complete this task or did so with grammatical errors and one paragraph.	
Discussion with Dr. Carlson	Student professionally communicated the situation and sought permission to grant an emergency appointment. *This grade is not based on the student's ability to sway the physician to allow an emergency appointment. It is based on student communication skills.*	N/A	N/A	Student failed to professionally communicate the situation and appropriately seek permission to grant an emergency appointment. *This grade is not based on the student's ability to sway the physician to allow an emergency appointment. It is based on student communication skills.*	

	Student correctly scheduled an appointment and obtained the required information with one or less errors.	Student correctly scheduled an appointment and obtained the required information with two errors.	Student correctly scheduled an appointment and obtained the required information with three to four errors.	Student failed to correctly schedule an appointment and/or failed to obtain the required information or did so with five or more errors.
Appointment Scheduling				
Schedule an Emergency Appointment Based on Approval	Student correctly scheduled an emergency appointment and obtained the required information with one or less errors.	Student correctly scheduled an emergency appointment and obtained the required information with two errors.	Student correctly scheduled an emergency appointment and obtained the required information with three to four errors.	Student failed to correctly schedule an emergency appointment and/or failed to obtain the required information or did so with five or more errors.
				TOTAL

Based on the above criteria the student's grade for this assignment is: _____

(Total the points for each element scored and average for a final grade.)

Comments to the Student:

Instructor Signature: _____ Date: _____

Third-Party Billing and Coding

Name _____ Date _____

Elements	4 Excellent	3 Proficient	2 Adequate	1 Needs Improvement	Points
Prepare Claim Form for Blue Cross/Blue Shield	Student correctly completed a claim form for Blue Cross/Blue Shield with one or less errors.	Student correctly completed a claim form for Blue Cross/Blue Shield with two errors.	Student correctly completed a claim form for Blue Cross/Blue Shield with three errors.	Student failed to correctly complete a claim form for Blue Cross/Blue Shield or did so with four or more errors.	
Sequence of Billing	Student appropriately explained the sequence of billing steps when submitting claims to third-party billers and Medicaid with one or less errors.	Student appropriately explained the sequence of billing steps when submitting claims to third-party billers and Medicaid with two errors.	Student appropriately explained the sequence of billing steps when submitting claims to third-party billers and Medicaid with three errors.	Student failed to appropriately explain the sequence of billing steps when submitting claims to third-party billers and Medicaid or did so with four or more errors.	
Identify Coding Errors	Student correctly identified the coding errors with no errors.	N/A	N/A	Student failed to correctly identify the coding errors or did so with errors.	
ICD-CM	Student demonstrated the ability to use the ICD-CM for billing and coding with no errors.	Student demonstrated the ability to use the ICD-CM for billing and coding with one error.	Student demonstrated the ability to use the ICD-CM for billing and coding with two errors.	Student failed to demonstrate the ability to use the ICD-CM for billing and coding or did so with three or more errors.	
CPT	Student demonstrated the ability to use the CPT for billing and coding with no errors.	Student demonstrated the ability to use the CPT for billing and coding with one error.	Student demonstrated the ability to use the CPT for billing and coding with two errors.	Student failed to demonstrate the ability to use the CPT for billing and coding or did so with three or more errors.	
Prepare Claim Form for Tricare	Student completed a corrected claim form to be submitted to Tricare with one or less errors.	Student completed a corrected claim form to be submitted to Tricare with two errors.	Student completed a corrected claim form to be submitted to Tricare with three errors.	Student failed to complete a corrected claim form for submittal to Tricare or did so with four or more errors.	
Relationship Between Procedure and Diagnostic Codes	Student accurately described the relationship between procedure and diagnostic codes with no errors.	N/A	N/A	Student failed to accurately describe the relationship between procedure and diagnostic codes or did so with errors.	

Description of Injuries	Student prepared a draft describing the patient's injuries with no errors.	Student prepared a draft describing the patient's injuries with one error.	Student prepared a draft describing the patient's injuries with two errors.	Student failed to prepare a draft describing the patient's injuries or did so with three or more errors.
Prepare Documents for Mail	Student correctly prepared the documents to be mailed with no errors.	N/A	N/A	Student failed to prepare the documents to be mailed or did so with errors.
				TOTAL

Based on the above criteria the student's grade for this assignment is: _____

(Total the points for each element scored and average for a final grade.)

Comments to the Student:

Instructor Signature: _____   Date: _____

Photocopier Maintenance and Repairs

Name _____ Date _____

Elements	4 Excellent	3 Proficient	2 Adequate	1 Needs Improvement	Points
Troubleshooting	Student provided a synopsis of possible causes for a paper jam.	N/A	N/A	Student failed to provide a synopsis of possible causes of a paper jam.	
Warranty	Student effectively determined whether required repairs will be covered or not.	N/A	N/A	Student failed to effectively determine whether required repairs will be covered or not.	
Repair Service	Student accurately located a company to service the photocopier.	N/A	N/A	Student failed to accurately locate a company to service the photocopier.	
Telephone Greeting and Introduction of Office and Self	Student appropriately greeted and introduced the office and self to the repair company with no errors.	Student appropriately greeted and introduced the office and self to the repair company with one error.	Student appropriately greeted and introduced the office and self to the repair company with two errors.	Student failed to appropriately greet and introduce the office and self to the repair company or did so with three or more errors.	
Appointment Scheduling	Student correctly scheduled an appointment and obtained the required information with no errors.	Students correctly scheduled an appointment and obtained the required information with one error.	Student correctly scheduled an appointment and obtained the required information with two errors.	Student failed to correctly schedule an appointment and/or failed to obtain the required information or did so with three or more errors.	
Routine Maintenance Scheduling	Student accurately established a routine maintenance schedule.	N/A	N/A	Student failed to accurately establish a routine maintenance schedule.	
Ending Telephone Calls	Student professionally ended the telephone call with no errors.	Student professionally ended the telephone call with one error.	Student professionally ended the telephone call with two errors.	Student professionally ended the telephone call with three or more errors or failed to professionally end the telephone call.	
				TOTAL	

Based on the above criteria the student's grade for this assignment is: _____

(Total the points for each element scored and average for a final grade.)

Comments to the Student:

Instructor Signature: _____ Date: _____

Office Equipment and Computer Concepts

Name _____ Date _____

Elements	4 Excellent	3 Proficient	2 Adequate	1 Needs Improvement	Points
Computer	Student reviewed and demonstrated computer usage with no errors.	Student reviewed and demonstrated computer usage with one error.	Student reviewed and demonstrated computer usage with two errors.	Student failed to review and demonstrate computer usage or did so with three or more errors.	
Calculator	Student reviewed and demonstrated calculator usage with no errors.	N/A	N/A	Student failed to review and demonstrate calculator usage or did so with errors.	
Scanner	Student reviewed and demonstrated scanner usage with no errors.	Student reviewed and demonstrated scanner usage with one error.	Student reviewed and demonstrated scanner usage with two errors.	Student failed to review and demonstrate scanner usage or did so with three or more errors.	
Copy Machine	Student reviewed and demonstrated copy machine usage with no errors.	Student reviewed and demonstrated copy machine usage with one error.	Student reviewed and demonstrated copy machine usage with two errors.	Student failed to review and demonstrate copy machine usage or did so with three or more errors.	
Fax Machine	Student reviewed and demonstrated fax machine usage with no errors.	Student reviewed and demonstrated fax machine usage with one error.	Student reviewed and demonstrated fax machine usage with two errors.	Student failed to review and demonstrate fax machine usage or did so with three or more errors.	
Printer	Student reviewed and demonstrated printer usage with no errors.	N/A	N/A	Student failed to review and demonstrate printer usage or did so with errors.	
Computer Components	Student demonstrated the use of various computer components with one or less errors.	Student demonstrated the use of various computer components with two errors.	Student demonstrated the use of various computer components with three errors.	Student failed to demonstrate the use of the various computer components or did so with four or more errors.	
Database Applications	Student reviewed and demonstrated database applications with one or less errors.	Student reviewed and demonstrated database applications with two errors.	Student reviewed and demonstrated database applications with three errors.	Student failed to review and demonstrate database applications or did so with four or more errors.	
Networks	Student reviewed and demonstrated network usage with no errors.	N/A	N/A	Student failed to review and demonstrate network usage or did so with errors.	

Security	Student reviewed and demonstrated security password applications with no errors.	N/A	N/A	Student failed to review and demonstrate security password applications or did so with errors.
Medical Management Software	Student reviewed and demonstrated medical practice management software usage with one or less errors.	Student reviewed and demonstrated medical practice management software usage with two to three errors.	Student reviewed and demonstrated medical practice management software usage with four to five errors.	Student failed to review and demonstrate medical practice management software usage or did so with six or more errors.
Extern Synopsis	Student completed an informative synopsis regarding his or her experience working with an extern.	N/A	N/A	Student failed to complete an informative synopsis regarding his or her experience working with an extern.
				TOTAL

Based on the above criteria the student's grade for this assignment is: _____

(Total the points for each element scored and average for a final grade.)

Comments to the Student:

Instructor Signature: _____   Date: _____

Scheduling Methods

Name _____   Date _____

Elements	4 Excellent	3 Proficient	2 Adequate	1 Needs Improvement	Points
Research Scheduling Methods	Student participated in researching scheduling methods.	N/A	N/A	Student failed to participate in researching scheduling methods.	
Description of Scheduling Methods	Student accurately described each scheduling method with no errors.	Student accurately described each scheduling method with one error.	Student accurately described each scheduling method with two errors.	Student failed to accurately describe each scheduling method or did so with three or more errors.	
Response to Question 3	Student appropriately stated the reasoning for his or her choice of scheduling methods.	N/A	N/A	Student failed to appropriately state the reasoning for his or her choice of scheduling methods or did so with errors.	
PowerPoint	Student created a professional PowerPoint presentation with no informational errors.	Student created a professional PowerPoint presentation with one informational error.	Student created a professional PowerPoint presentation with two informational errors.	Student failed to create a professional PowerPoint presentation or did so with three or more informational errors.	
Presentation	Student professionally presented his or her PowerPoint presentation and choice of scheduling methods.	N/A	N/A	Student failed to professionally present a PowerPoint presentation and choice of scheduling methods.	
				TOTAL	

Based on the above criteria the student's grade for this assignment is: _____
(Total the points for each element scored and average for a final grade.)

Comments to the Student:

Instructor Signature: _____   Date: _____

CASE STUDY 20 *Managing an Angry Caller*

Name _____ Date _____

Elements	4 Excellent	3 Proficient	2 Adequate	1 Needs Improvement	Points
Telephone Greeting and Introduction of Office and Self	Student appropriately greeted and introduced the office and self to the patient with one or less errors.	Student appropriately greeted and introduced the office and self to the patient with two errors.	Student appropriately greeted and introduced the office and self to the patient with three to four errors.	Student failed to appropriately greet and introduce the office and self to the patient or did so with five or more errors.	
Demonstrating Multiple-Line Competency	Student demonstrated competency in this skill with one or less errors.	Student demonstrated competency in this skill with two errors.	Student demonstrated competency in this skill with three to four errors.	Student failed to demonstrate competency in this skill or did so with five or more errors.	
Telephone Call Screening	Student accurately screened all five telephone calls.	Student accurately screened four telephone calls.	Student accurately screened three telephone calls.	Student accurately screened one to two telephone calls or failed to screen any telephone calls.	
Gathering Data over the Telephone with Patient Interview/ Questioning Techniques	Student gathered pertinent patient data while using interview/questioning techniques with no errors.	Student gathered pertinent patient data while using interview/questioning techniques with one to two errors.	Student gathered pertinent patient data while using interview/questioning techniques with three to four errors.	Student gathered pertinent patient data while using interview/questioning techniques with five or more errors or failed to gather pertinent information from the patient.	
Evaluating the Effectiveness of Patient Interviewing Techniques	Student employed observational and active listening skills and provided appropriate feedback with one or less errors.	Student employed observational and active listening skills and provided appropriate feedback with two errors.	Student employed observational and active listening skills and provided appropriate feedback with three to four errors.	Student employed observational and active listening skills and provided appropriate feedback with five or more errors.	
Angry Caller	Student appropriately handled an angry caller.	N/A	N/A	Student failed to appropriately handle an angry caller.	
Ending Telephone Calls	Student professionally ended all telephone calls with one or less errors.	Student professionally ended all telephone calls with two errors.	Student professionally ended all telephone calls with three errors.	Student professionally ended all telephone calls with four or more errors or failed to professionally end any telephone calls.	
Written Response	Student appropriately responded to all seven questions.	Student appropriately responded to six questions.	Student appropriately responded to five questions.	Student failed to appropriately respond to four or less questions or failed to respond to any of the questions.	
				TOTAL	

Based on the above criteria the student's grade for this assignment is: _____

(Total the points for each element scored and average for a final grade.)

Comments to the Student:

Instructor Signature: _____ Date: _____

HIPAA—Privacy and Breach of Confidentiality

Name _____ Date _____

Elements	4 Excellent	3 Proficient	2 Adequate	1 Needs Improvement	Points
Response to Question 1	Student responded appropriately to question 1 with one or less errors.	Student responded appropriately to question 1 with two errors.	Student responded appropriately to question 1 with three errors.	Student failed to respond appropriately to question 1 or did so with four or more errors.	
Response to Question 2	Student responded appropriately to question 2 with one or less errors.	Student responded appropriately to question 2 with two errors.	Student responded appropriately to question 2 with three errors.	Student failed to respond appropriately to question 2 or did so with four or more errors.	
Response to Question 3	Student responded appropriately to question 3 with no errors.	Student responded appropriately to question 3 with one error.	Student responded appropriately to question 3 with two errors.	Student failed to respond appropriately to question 3 or did so with three or more errors.	
Response to Question 4	Student responded appropriately to question 4 with one or less errors.	Student responded appropriately to question 4 with two errors.	Student responded appropriately to question 4 with three errors.	Student failed to respond appropriately to question 4 or did so with four or more errors.	
Role-Play	Student participated in the role-play scenario.	N/A	N/A	Student failed to participate in the role-play scenario.	
Displaying a Professional Attitude and Communication Skills	Student displayed a professional attitude and communication skills during the role-play.	N/A	N/A	Student failed to display a professional attitude and communication skills during the role-play.	
Accepting Responsibility	Student discussed accepting responsibility during the role-play.	N/A	N/A	Student failed to discuss accepting responsibility during the role-play.	
Supporting the Professional Organization	Student competently discussed the need for the staff to support the professional organization during the role-play.	N/A	N/A	Student failed to competently discuss the need for the staff to support the professional organization during the role-play or discussed it without efficiently supporting the need.	
Promoting Patient Care	Student addressed the effect of Marcy's actions on promoting competent patient care.	N/A	N/A	Student failed to address the effect of Marcy's actions on promoting competent patient care.	

Use Tact, Diplomacy, and Integrity	Student appropriately discussed how to handle the situation using tact, diplomacy, and integrity.			Student failed to appropriately discuss how to handle the situation using tact, diplomacy, and integrity.
Fundamental Writing Skills	Student appropriately used medical terminology, sentence structure, grammar, and punctuation with one or less errors.	Student appropriately used medical terminology, sentence structure, grammar, and punctuation with two errors.	Student appropriately used medical terminology, sentence structure, grammar, and punctuation with three errors.	Student failed to appropriately use medical terminology, sentence structure, grammar, and punctuation or did so with four or more errors.
Letter	Student correctly formatted a letter with one or less errors.	Student correctly formatted a letter with two errors.	Student correctly formatted a letter with three errors.	Student failed to correctly format a letter or did so with four or more errors.
Electronic Mail	Student submitted his or her letter via e-mail.	N/A	N/A	Student failed to submit his or her letter via e-mail.
				TOTAL

Based on the above criteria the student's grade for this assignment is: _____

(Total the points for each element scored and average for a final grade.)

Comments to the Student:

Instructor Signature: _____   Date: _____

Research and Memo for CLIA and Point-of-Care Testing

Name _____ Date _____

Elements	4 Excellent	3 Proficient	2 Adequate	1 Needs Improvement	Points
Internet Search	Student correctly performed an Internet search and located CLIA guidelines regarding point-of-care tests and CLIA-waived tests with one or less errors.	Student correctly performed an Internet search and located CLIA guidelines regarding point-of-care tests and CLIA-waived tests with two errors.	Student correctly performed an Internet search and located CLIA guidelines regarding point-of-care tests and CLIA-waived tests with three errors.	Student failed to correctly perform an Internet search or did not locate correct information or did so with four or more errors.	
Fundamental Writing Skills	Student appropriately used medical terminology, sentence structure, grammar, and punctuation with one or less errors.	Student appropriately used medical terminology, sentence structure, grammar, and punctuation with two errors.	Student appropriately used medical terminology, sentence structure, grammar, and punctuation with three errors.	Student failed to appropriately use medical terminology, sentence structure, grammar, and punctuation or did so with four or more errors.	
Memo	Student appropriately used the MLA or APA format for citing sources within the memo with no errors.	Student appropriately used the MLA or APA format for citing sources within the memo with one error.	Student appropriately used the MLA or APA format for citing sources within the memo with two errors.	Student failed to appropriately use the MLA or APA format for citing sources or did so with three or more errors.	
Proofreading	Student implemented the required changes in the final draft of his or her proofread memo.	N/A	N/A	Student failed to implement the required changes to the final draft of his or her proofread memo.	
Electronic Mail	Student submitted the memo via e-mail.	N/A	N/A	Student failed to submit the memo via e-mail.	
				TOTAL	

Based on the above criteria the student's grade for this assignment is: _____

(Total the points for each element scored and average for a final grade.)

Comments to the Student:

Instructor Signature: _____ Date: _____

CASE STUDY 23   *Pre-Op Consultation*

Name _____   Date _____

Elements	4 Excellent	3 Proficient	2 Adequate	1 Needs Improvement	Points
Obtain Patient Chart	Student obtained the patient's chart.	N/A	N/A	Student failed to obtain the patient's chart.	
Introduction to Patient	Student appropriately introduced self to the patient with no errors.	N/A	N/A	Student failed to appropriately introduce self to the patient or did so with errors.	
Scheduling a Lumpectomy	Student appropriately scheduled a lumpectomy with no errors.	N/A	N/A	Student failed to appropriately schedule a lumpectomy or did so with errors.	
Appointment Card and Procedural Instructions	Student provided the patient with an appointment card and procedural instructions with no errors.	Student provided the patient with an appointment card and procedural instructions with one error.	Student provided the patient with an appointment card and procedural instructions with three errors.	Student failed to provide the patient with an appointment card and procedural instructions or did so with four or more errors.	
Medicare Preauthorization and Precertification	Student correctly performed a Medicare preauthorization and precertification with one or less errors.	Student correctly performed a Medicare preauthorization and precertification with two errors.	Student correctly performed a Medicare preauthorization and precertification with three errors.	Student failed to correctly perform a Medicare preauthorization and precertification or did so with four or more errors.	
Pre-Op Consultation	Student accurately performed a pre-op consultation with the patient with one or less errors.	Student accurately performed a pre-op consultation with the patient with two errors.	Student accurately performed a pre-op consultation with the patient with three errors.	Student failed to accurately perform a pre-op consultation with the patient or did so with four or more errors.	
Insurance Card	Student obtained a copy of the patient's insurance card.	N/A	N/A	Student failed to obtain a copy of the patient's insurance card.	
Consent Forms	Student obtained the appropriate consent forms.	N/A	N/A	Student failed to obtain the appropriate consent forms.	
Fax	Student faxed the appropriate information to Dr. Robinson's office.	N/A	N/A	Student failed to fax the appropriate information to Dr. Robinson's office.	
Referral Call and Response to Question 10	Student appropriately called the oncologist and answered the question properly with one or less errors.	Student appropriately called the oncologist and answered the question properly with two errors.	Student appropriately called the oncologist and answered the question properly with three errors.	Student failed to appropriately call the oncologist and answer the question properly or did so with four or more errors.	
				TOTAL	

Based on the above criteria the student's grade for this assignment is: _____
(Total the points for each element scored and average for a final grade.)

Comments to the Student:

Instructor Signature: _____ Date: _____

Breach of Confidentiality–Intentional Tort

Name _____ Date _____

Elements	4 Excellent	3 Proficient	2 Adequate	1 Needs Improvement	Points
PowerPoint Presentation	Student submitted a 10–12 slide presentation.	Student submitted an eight to nine slide presentation.	Student submitted a six to seven slide presentation.	Student failed to submit a slide presentation or did so with five slides or less.	
Fundamental Writing Skills	Student appropriately used medical terminology, sentence structure, grammar, and punctuation with one or less errors.	Student appropriately used medical terminology, sentence structure, grammar, and punctuation with two errors.	Student appropriately used medical terminology, sentence structure, grammar, and punctuation with three errors.	Student failed to appropriately use medical terminology, sentence structure, grammar, and punctuation or did so with four or more errors.	
Medical Practice Acts	Student addressed medical practice acts in the PowerPoint presentation.	N/A	N/A	Student failed to address medical practice acts in the PowerPoint presentation.	
Physician-Patient Relationship	Student addressed a physician-patient relationship and the impact that an impending lawsuit will have on that relationship.	N/A	N/A	Student failed to address a physician-patient relationship and the impact that an impending lawsuit will have on that relationship or only addressed a physician-patient relationship.	
Responsibility and Rights of a Patient, Physician, and Medical Assistant	Student addressed the responsibility and rights of all three individuals with one or less errors.	Student addressed the responsibility and rights of all three individuals with two errors.	Student addressed the responsibility and rights of all three individuals with three errors.	Student failed to address the responsibility and rights of all three individuals or did so with four or more errors.	
Professional Liability	Student correctly addressed professional liability with no errors.	Student correctly addressed professional liability with one error.	Student correctly addressed professional liability with two errors.	Student failed to correctly address professional liability or did so with three or more errors.	
Maintaining Confidentiality	Student addressed maintaining confidentiality and its impact on lawsuits.	N/A	N/A	Student failed to address maintaining confidentiality and its impact on lawsuits or only addressed maintaining confidentiality and neglected to address its impact on lawsuits.	
Intentional Tort: Invasion of Privacy, Slander, and Libel	Student addressed all three intentional torts with one or less errors.	Student addressed all three intentional torts with two errors.	Student addressed all three intentional torts with three errors.	Student failed to address all three intentional torts or did so with four or more errors.	

Ethics	Student addressed the role of ethics in the current situation in his or her PowerPoint presentation.	N/A	Student failed to address the role of ethics in the current situation in his or her PowerPoint presentation.	
Electronic Mail	Student submitted his or her letter via e-mail.	N/A	Student failed to submit his or her letter via e-mail.	
			TOTAL	

Based on the above criteria the student's grade for this assignment is: _____

(Total the points for each element scored and average for a final grade.)

Comments to the Student:

Instructor Signature: _____   Date: _____

CASE STUDY 25 *Termination of Employment*

Name _____ Date _____

Elements	4 Excellent	3 Proficient	2 Adequate	1 Needs Improvement	Points
Role-Play Scenario 1	Student participated in the role-play scenario between Dr. Carlson and Barbara with one or less errors.	Student participated in the role-play scenario between Dr. Carlson and Barbara with two errors.	Student participated in the role-play scenario between Dr. Carlson and Barbara with three to four errors.	Student failed to participate in the role-play scenario between Dr. Carlson and Barbara or did so with five or more errors.	
Response to Question 2	Student responded appropriately to question 2 with one or less errors.	Student responded appropriately to question 2 with two errors.	Student responded appropriately to question 2 with three to four errors.	Student failed to respond appropriately to question 2 or did so with five or more errors.	
Response to Question 3	Student responded appropriately to question 3 with one or less errors.	Student responded appropriately to question 3 with two errors.	Student responded appropriately to question 3 with three to four errors.	Student failed to respond appropriately to question 3 or did so with five or more errors.	
Response to Question 4	Student responded appropriately to question 4 with one or less errors.	Student responded appropriately to question 4 with two errors.	Student responded appropriately to question 4 with three to four errors.	Student failed to respond appropriately to question 4 or did so with five or more errors.	
Response to Question 5	Student responded appropriately to question 5 with one or less errors.	Student responded appropriately to question 5 with two errors.	Student responded appropriately to question 5 with three to four errors.	Student failed to respond appropriately to question 5 or did so with five or more errors.	
Response to Question 6	Student responded appropriately to question 6 with one or less errors.	Student responded appropriately to question 6 with two errors.	Student responded appropriately to question 6 with three to four errors.	Student failed to respond appropriately to question 6 or did so with five or more errors.	
Response to Question 7	Student responded appropriately to question 7 with one or less errors.	Student responded appropriately to question 7 with two errors.	Student responded appropriately to question 7 with three to four errors.	Student failed to respond appropriately to question 7 or did so with five or more errors.	
Role-Play Scenario 2	Student participated in the role-play scenario between Dr. Carlson and Angie with one or less errors.	Student participated in the role-play scenario between Dr. Carlson and Angie with two errors.	Student participated in the role-play scenario between Dr. Carlson and Angie with three to four errors.	Student failed to participate in the role-play scenario between Dr. Carlson and Angie or did so with five or more errors.	

Observation and Synopsis of Verbal and Nonverbal Communication	Student participated in observing classmates during role-play scenario 2 and wrote a one-paragraph synopsis evaluating the verbal and nonverbal communication with one or less errors.	Student participated in observing classmates during role-play scenario 2 and wrote a one-paragraph synopsis evaluating the verbal and nonverbal communication with two errors.	Student participated in observing classmates during role-play scenario 2 and wrote a one-paragraph synopsis evaluating the verbal and nonverbal communication with three to four errors.	Student failed to participate in observing classmates during role-play scenario 2 and/or did not write a one-paragraph synopsis evaluating the verbal and nonverbal communication or did so with five or more errors.
Employment Policy and Procedure Manual Entry	Student created an entry for the clinic's employment policy and procedure manual outlining the grounds for termination, specifically addressing "Breach of Confidentiality," with one or less errors.	Student created an entry for the clinic's employment policy and procedure manual outlining the grounds for termination, specifically addressing "Breach of Confidentiality," with two errors.	Student created an entry for the clinic's employment policy and procedure manual outlining the grounds for termination, specifically addressing "Breach of Confidentiality," with three to four errors.	Student failed to create an entry for the clinic's employment policy and procedure manual outlining the grounds for termination, specifically addressing "Breach of Confidentiality," or did so with five or more errors.
				TOTAL

Based on the above criteria the student's grade for this assignment is: _____

(Total the points for each element scored and average for a final grade.)

Comments to the Student:

Instructor Signature: _____ Date: _____

Informational Report–FDA Guidelines

Name _____ Date _____

Elements	4 Excellent	3 Proficient	2 Adequate	1 Needs Improvement	Points
Internet Search	Student correctly performed an Internet search and located FDA guidelines pertinent to the functioning of the clinic with one or less errors.	Student correctly performed an Internet search and located FDA guidelines pertinent to the functioning of the clinic with two errors.	Student correctly performed an Internet search and located FDA guidelines pertinent to the functioning of the clinic with three errors.	Student failed to correctly perform an Internet search to locate FDA guidelines pertinent to the functioning of the clinic or did so with four or more errors.	
Fundamental Writing Skills	Student appropriately used medical terminology, sentence structure, grammar, and punctuation with one or less errors.	Student appropriately used medical terminology, sentence structure, grammar, and punctuation with two errors.	Student appropriately used medical terminology, sentence structure, grammar, and punctuation with three errors.	Student failed to appropriately use medical terminology, sentence structure, grammar, and punctuation or did so with four or more errors.	
Report	Student appropriately used the MLA or APA format for report writing and correctly cited the source articles with one or less errors.	Student appropriately used the MLA or APA format for report writing and correctly cited the source articles with two errors.	Student appropriately used the MLA or APA format for report writing and correctly cited the source articles with three to four errors.	Student failed to appropriately use the MLA or APA format for report writing and correctly cite the source articles or did so with five or more errors.	
Report Requirements	Student submitted a two-page report.	Student submitted a one-and-a-half-page report.	Student submitted a one-page report.	Student failed to submit a report or submitted one-half page or less.	
Report Proofreading	Student applied appropriate proofreading techniques and marks to his or her classmate's report with one or less errors.	Student applied appropriate proofreading techniques and marks to his or her classmate's report with two errors.	Student applied appropriate proofreading techniques and marks to his or her classmate's report with three errors.	Student failed to apply appropriate proofreading techniques and marks to his or her classmate's report or did so with four or more errors.	
Constructive Criticism and Evaluation	Student provided constructive criticism and an honest evaluation of his or her classmate's report.	N/A	N/A	Student failed to provide constructive criticism or an honest evaluation of his or her classmate's report.	
Oral Presentation	Student applied professional communication skills during oral presentation.	N/A	N/A	Student failed to apply professional communication skills during oral presentation.	
				TOTAL	

Based on the above criteria the student's grade for this assignment is: _____

(Total the points for each element scored and average for a final grade.)

Comments to the Student:

Instructor Signature: _____ Date: _____

Medical Liability Coverage

Name _____ Date _____

Elements	4 Excellent	3 Proficient	2 Adequate	1 Needs Improvement	Points
Internet Search	Student correctly performed an Internet search and located current information on medical liability coverage dated within the past six months.	N/A	N/A	Student failed to correctly perform an Internet search or did not locate current information on medical liability coverage dated within the past six months.	
Types and Rates for Coverage	Student successfully located three types of medical liability coverage including rates.	Student successfully located two types of medical liability coverage including rates.	Student successfully located one type of medical liability coverage including rate.	Student failed to successfully locate any type of medical liability coverage or rates.	
Fundamental Writing Skills	Student appropriately used medical terminology, sentence structure, grammar, and punctuation with one or less errors.	Student appropriately used medical terminology, sentence structure, grammar, and punctuation with two errors.	Student appropriately used medical terminology, sentence structure, grammar, and punctuation with three errors.	Student failed to appropriately use medical terminology, sentence structure, grammar, and punctuation or did so with four or more errors.	
Spreadsheet	Student successfully created a spreadsheet containing medical liability coverage information with one or less errors.	Student successfully created a spreadsheet containing medical liability coverage information with two errors.	Student successfully created a spreadsheet containing medical liability coverage information with three errors.	Student failed to successfully create a spreadsheet containing medical liability coverage information or did so with four or more errors.	
Graph	Student created a graph within the spreadsheet that compared and contrasted the types of coverage available.	N/A	N/A	Student failed to create a graph within the spreadsheet that compared and contrasted the types of coverage available.	
Saving to a Flash Drive	Student successfully saved the spreadsheet to a flash drive.	N/A	N/A	Student failed to save the spreadsheet to a flash drive.	
				TOTAL	

Based on the above criteria the student's grade for this assignment is: _____

(Total the points for each element scored and average for a final grade.)

Comments to the Student:

Instructor Signature: _____ Date: _____

ADA—Wheelchair Accessibility

Name _____ Date _____

Elements	4 Excellent	3 Proficient	2 Adequate	1 Needs Improvement	Points
Internet Search	Student correctly performed an Internet search and located the requirements for wheelchair accessibility dated within the past six months with one or less errors.	Student correctly performed an Internet search and located the requirements for wheelchair accessibility dated within the past six months with two errors.	Student correctly performed an Internet search and located the requirements for wheelchair accessibility dated within the past six months with three errors.	Student failed to correctly perform an Internet search or did not locate the requirements for wheelchair accessibility dated within the past six months or did so with four or more errors.	
Fundamental Writing Skills	Student appropriately used medical terminology, sentence structure, grammar, and punctuation with one or less errors.	Student appropriately used medical terminology, sentence structure, grammar, and punctuation with two errors.	Student appropriately used medical terminology, sentence structure, grammar, and punctuation with three errors.	Student failed to appropriately use medical terminology, sentence structure, grammar, and punctuation or did so with four or more errors.	
Report	Student appropriately used the MLA or APA format for report writing and correctly cited the source articles with one or less errors.	Student appropriately used the MLA or APA format for report writing and correctly cited the source articles with two errors.	Student appropriately used the MLA or APA format for report writing and correctly cited the source articles with three to four errors.	Student failed to appropriately use the MLA or APA format for report writing and to correctly cite the source articles or did so with five or more errors.	
Electronic Mail	Student submitted the report via e-mail.	N/A	N/A	Student failed to submit the report via e-mail.	
Measurement of Doorways and Hallways	Student demonstrated the ability to correctly measure the doorways and hallways with no errors.	Student demonstrated the ability to correctly measure doorways and hallways with one error.	Student demonstrated the ability to correctly measure doorways and hallways with two errors.	Student failed to demonstrate the ability to measure doorways and hallways or did so with three or more errors.	
Research Cost for Implementing ADA Requirements	Student researched the cost for implementing ADA requirements.	N/A	N/A	Student failed to research the cost for implementing ADA requirements.	
Response to Question 5	Student answered the question properly with one or less errors.	Student answered the question properly with two errors.	Student answered the question properly with three errors.	Student failed to answer the question properly or did so with four or more errors.	
Liability for Noncompliance to ADA Guidelines	Student accurately reported the clinic's liability for noncompliance to ADA guidelines.	N/A	N/A	Student failed to accurately report the clinic's liability for noncompliance to ADA guidelines.	
				TOTAL	

Based on the above criteria the student's grade for this assignment is: _____

(Total the points for each element scored and average for a final grade.)

Comments to the Student:

Instructor Signature: _____ Date: _____

Patient Education, Community Support Groups, Stages of Grief

Name _____ Date _____

Elements	4 Excellent	3 Proficient	2 Adequate	1 Needs Improvement	Points
Role-Play Scenario 1	Student participated in the role-play scenario between Angie and the medical assistant with one or less errors.	Student participated in the role-play scenario between Angie and the medical assistant with two errors.	Student participated in the role-play scenario between Angie and the medical assistant with three to four errors.	Student failed to participate in the role-play scenario between Angie and the medical assistant or did so with five or more errors.	
Comforted Angie and Listened to Her Concerns	Student responded appropriately to step 1a with one or less errors.	Student responded appropriately to step 1a with two errors.	Student responded appropriately to step 1a with three to four errors.	Student failed to respond appropriately to step 1a or did so with five or more errors.	
Explanation of the Grief Process	Student responded appropriately to step 1b with one or less errors.	Student responded appropriately to step 1b with two errors.	Student responded appropriately to step 1b with three to four errors.	Student failed to respond appropriately to step 1b or did so with five or more errors.	
Explanation of HIV	Student responded appropriately to step 1c with one or less errors.	Student responded appropriately to step 1c with two errors.	Student responded appropriately to step 1c with three to four errors.	Student failed to respond appropriately to step 1c or did so with five or more errors.	
Community Support Groups	Student responded appropriately to step 1d with one or less errors.	Student responded appropriately to step 1d with two errors.	Student responded appropriately to step 1d with three to four errors.	Student failed to respond appropriately to step 1d or did so with five or more errors.	
Response to Question 2	Student responded appropriately to question 2 with one or less errors.	Student responded appropriately to question 2 with two errors.	Student responded appropriately to question 2 with three to four errors.	Student failed to respond appropriately to question 2 or did so with five or more errors.	
Documentation	Student properly documented with one or less errors.	Student properly documented with two errors.	Student properly documented with three to four errors.	Student failed to properly document or did so with five or more errors.	
				TOTAL	

Based on the above criteria the student's grade for this assignment is: _____

(Total the points for each element scored and average for a final grade.)

Comments to the Student:

Instructor Signature: _____ Date: _____

Policy and Procedure Manual and Notification Letter

Name _____   Date _____

Elements	4 Excellent	3 Proficient	2 Adequate	1 Needs Improvement	Points
Document for Policy and Procedure Manual	Student compiled information onto a professional document with one or less errors.	Student compiled information onto a professional document with two errors.	Student compiled information onto a professional document with three errors.	Student failed to compile information onto a professional document or did so with four or more errors.	
Watermark	Student correctly placed a watermark on the document.	N/A	N/A	Student failed to correctly place a watermark on the document.	
Fundamental Writing Skills of Document	Student appropriately used medical terminology, sentence structure, grammar, and punctuation with one or less errors.	Student appropriately used medical terminology, sentence structure, grammar, and punctuation with two errors.	Student appropriately used medical terminology, sentence structure, grammar, and punctuation with three errors.	Student failed to appropriately use medical terminology, sentence structure, grammar, and punctuation or did so with four or more errors.	
Proofreading	Student implemented the required changes to the final draft of the proofread document.	N/A	N/A	Student failed to implement the required changes to the final draft of the proofread document.	
Letter	Student correctly formatted a formal letter of notification with one or less errors.	Student correctly formatted a formal letter of notification with two errors.	Student correctly formatted a formal letter of notification with three errors.	Student failed to correctly format a formal letter of notification or did so with four or more errors.	
Fundamental Writing Skills of Letter	Student appropriately used medical terminology, sentence structure, grammar, and punctuation with one or less errors.	Student appropriately used medical terminology, sentence structure, grammar, and punctuation with two errors.	Student appropriately used medical terminology, sentence structure, grammar, and punctuation with three errors.	Student failed to appropriately use medical terminology, sentence structure, grammar, and punctuation or did so with four or more errors.	
Preparing Letters and Envelopes	Student correctly prepared the letters and envelopes, following postal guidelines for outgoing mail, with one or less errors.	Student correctly prepared the letters and envelopes, following postal guidelines for outgoing mail, with two errors.	Student correctly prepared the letters and envelopes, following postal guidelines for outgoing mail, with three errors.	Student failed to correctly prepare the letters and envelopes, following postal guidelines for outgoing mail, or did so with four or more errors.	
Postal Machine/ Meter	Student demonstrated the ability to use a postal machine/meter.	N/A	N/A	Student failed to demonstrate the ability to use a postal machine/meter.	
				TOTAL	

Based on the above criteria the student's grade for this assignment is: _____
(Total the points for each element scored and average for a final grade.)

Comments to the Student:

Instructor Signature: _____ Date: _____

OSHA–Biohazardous Waste Research and Report

Name _____ Date _____

Elements	4 Excellent	3 Proficient	2 Adequate	1 Needs Improvement	Points
Internet Search	Student correctly performed an Internet search and located the requirements for the disposal of biohazardous waste, dated within the past six months, with one or less errors.	Student correctly performed an Internet search and located the requirements for the disposal of biohazardous waste, dated within the past six months, with two errors.	Student correctly performed an Internet search and located the requirements for the disposal of biohazardous waste, dated within the past six months, with three to four errors.	Student failed to correctly perform an Internet search or did not locate the requirements for the disposal of biohazardous waste, dated within the past six months, or did so with five or more errors.	
Report Word Requirements	Student submitted a report with 1,000 words or more.	Student submitted a report with 950–999 words.	Student submitted a report with 900–949 words.	Student failed to submit a report or did so with less than 900 words.	
Fundamental Writing Skills	Student appropriately used medical terminology, sentence structure, grammar, and punctuation with one or less errors.	Student appropriately used medical terminology, sentence structure, grammar, and punctuation with two errors.	Student appropriately used medical terminology, sentence structure, grammar, and punctuation with three to four errors.	Student failed to appropriately use medical terminology, sentence structure, grammar, and punctuation or did so with five or more errors.	
Ideas for Implementing Updates	Student submitted three ideas for implementing OSHA updates to the clinic.	Student submitted two ideas for implementing OSHA updates to the clinic.	Student submitted one idea for implementing OSHA updates to the clinic.	Student failed to submit ideas for implementing OSHA updates to the clinic.	
Report	Student appropriately used the MLA or APA format for report writing and correctly cited the source articles with one or less errors.	Student appropriately used the MLA or APA format for report writing and correctly cited the source articles with two errors.	Student appropriately used the MLA or APA format for report writing and correctly cited the source articles with three to four errors.	Student failed to appropriately use the MLA or APA format for report writing and to correctly cite the source articles or did so with five or more errors.	
				TOTAL	

Based on the above criteria the student's grade for this assignment is: _____
(Total the points for each element scored and average for a final grade.)

Comments to the Student:

Instructor Signature: _____ Date: _____

CASE STUDY 32   *OSHA–Office Memo*

Name _____   Date _____

Elements	4 Excellent	3 Proficient	2 Adequate	1 Needs Improvement	Points
Memo Word Requirements	Student submitted a memo with 300 words or more.	Student submitted a memo with 275–299 words.	Student submitted a memo with 250–274 words.	Student failed to submit a memo or did so with less than 250 words.	
Fundamental Writing Skills	Student appropriately used medical terminology, sentence structure, grammar, and punctuation with one or less errors.	Student appropriately used medical terminology, sentence structure, grammar, and punctuation with two errors.	Student appropriately used medical terminology, sentence structure, grammar, and punctuation with three to four errors.	Student failed to appropriately use medical terminology, sentence structure, grammar, and punctuation or did so with five or more errors.	
Memo	Student appropriately used the MLA or APA format for memo writing and correctly cited the source articles with one or less errors.	Student appropriately used the MLA or APA format for memo writing and correctly cited the source articles with two errors.	Student appropriately used the MLA or APA format for memo writing and correctly cited the source articles with three to four errors.	Student failed to appropriately use the MLA or APA format for memo writing and to correctly cite the source articles or did so with five or more errors.	
Question Submission	Student submitted an appropriate response to each of the five questions.	Student submitted an appropriate response to four questions.	Student submitted an appropriate response to three questions.	Student failed to submit an appropriate response to the questions or did so to less than three questions.	
				TOTAL	

Based on the above criteria the student's grade for this assignment is: _____

(Total the points for each element scored and average for a final grade.)

Comments to the Student:

Instructor Signature: _____   Date: _____

Wellness Physical Examination, Patient Assessment

Name _____ Date _____

Elements	4 Excellent	3 Proficient	2 Adequate	1 Needs Improvement	Points
New-Patient Chart	Student correctly assembled a new-patient chart and completed all forms with one or less errors.	Student correctly assembled a new-patient chart and completed all forms with two errors.	Student correctly assembled a new-patient chart and completed all forms with three to four errors.	Student failed to correctly assemble a new-patient chart and/or failed to complete all forms or did so with five or more errors.	
Medical Asepsis and Standard Precautions	Student correctly performed medical aseptic techniques and observed all required standard precautions with one or less errors.	Student correctly performed medical aseptic techniques and observed all required standard precautions with two errors.	Student correctly performed medical aseptic techniques and observed all required standard precautions with three to four errors.	Student failed to correctly perform medical aseptic techniques and observe all required standard precautions or did so with five or more errors.	
Introduction to Patient	Student appropriately introduced self to the patient with one or less errors.	Student appropriately introduced self to the patient with two errors.	Student appropriately introduced self to the patient with three to four errors.	Student failed to appropriately introduce self to the patient or did so with five or more errors.	
Obtained Intake Information	Student appropriately obtained patient intake information with one or less errors.	Student appropriately obtained patient intake information with two errors.	Student appropriately obtained patient intake information with three to four errors.	Student failed to appropriately obtain patient intake information or did so with five or more errors.	
Explanation of Procedure(s)	Student appropriately explained the procedure(s) to the patient with one or less errors.	Student appropriately explained the procedure(s) to the patient with two errors.	Student appropriately explained the procedure(s) to the patient with three to four errors.	Student failed to appropriately explain the procedure(s) to the patient or did so with five or more errors.	
Patient Assessment • Height	Student performed a full patient assessment with one to two errors.	Student performed a full patient assessment with two to three errors or omitted one skill assessment.	Student performed a full patient assessment with four to five errors or omitted two skill assessments.	Student performed a full patient assessment with six or more errors or omitted three or more skills.	
Patient Assessment • Weight	Student performed a full patient assessment with one to two errors.	Student performed a full patient assessment with two to three errors or omitted one skill assessment.	Student performed a full patient assessment with four to five errors or omitted two skill assessments.	Student performed a full patient assessment with six or more errors or omitted three or more skills.	
Patient Assessment • Temperature	Student performed a full patient assessment with one to two errors.	Student performed a full patient assessment with two to three errors or student omitted one skill assessment.	Student performed a full patient assessment with four to five errors or student omitted two skill assessments.	Student performed a full patient assessment with six or more errors or student omitted three or more skills.	

Criteria				
Patient Assessment • Pulse	Student performed a full patient assessment with one to two errors.	Student performed a full patient assessment with two to three errors or omitted one skill assessment.	Student performed a full patient assessment with four to five errors or omitted two skill assessments.	Student performed a full patient assessment with six or more errors or omitted three or more skills.
Patient Assessment • Respiration	Student performed a full patient assessment with one to two errors.	Student performed a full patient assessment with two to three errors or omitted one skill assessment.	Student performed a full patient assessment with four to five errors or omitted two skill assessments.	Student performed a full patient assessment with six or more errors or omitted three or more skills.
Patient Assessment • Blood Pressure	Student performed a full patient assessment with one to two errors.	Student performed a full patient assessment with two to three errors or omitted one skill assessment.	Student performed a full patient assessment with four to five errors or omitted two skill assessments.	Student performed a full patient assessment with six or more errors or omitted three or more skills.
Patient Instructions	Student provided appropriate patient instruction with one or less errors.	Student provided appropriate patient instruction with two errors.	Student provided appropriate patient instruction with three to four errors.	Student failed to provide appropriate patient instruction or did so with five or more errors.
Position and Draping	Student properly positioned and draped the patient for a routine physical examination with one or less errors.	Student properly positioned and draped the patient for a routine physical examination with two errors.	Student properly positioned and draped the patient for a routine physical examination with three to four errors.	Student failed to properly position and drape the patient or did so with five or more errors or positioned and draped the patient for the incorrect procedure.
Documentation	Student properly documented all procedures with one or less errors.	Student properly documented procedures with two errors or omitted documentation of one procedure.	Student properly documented procedures with three to four errors or omitted documentation of two procedures.	Student properly documented procedures with five or more errors or omitted documentation of three or more procedures.
Supplies and Equipment	Student provided the physician with the appropriate supplies and equipment with one or less errors.	Student provided the physician with the appropriate supplies and equipment with two errors.	Student provided the physician with the appropriate supplies and equipment with three to four errors.	Student failed to provide the appropriate supplies and equipment or did so with six or more errors.
				TOTAL

Based on the above criteria the student's grade for this assignment is: _____

(Total the points for each element scored and average for a final grade.)

Comments to the Student:

Instructor Signature: _____   Date: _____

Patient Education, Patient Assessment

Name _____ Date _____

Elements	4 Excellent	3 Proficient	2 Adequate	1 Needs Improvement	Points
Medical Asepsis and Standard Precautions	Student correctly performed medical aseptic techniques and observed all required standard precautions with one or less errors.	Student correctly performed medical aseptic techniques and observed all required standard precautions with two errors.	Student correctly performed medical aseptic techniques and observed all required standard precautions with three to four errors.	Student failed to correctly perform medical aseptic techniques and observe all required standard precautions or did so with five or more errors.	
Supplies and Equipment	Student obtained and had available appropriate supplies and equipment with one or less errors.	Student obtained and had available supplies and equipment with two errors.	Student obtained and had available supplies and equipment with three to four errors.	Student failed to obtain or have available supplies and equipment or did so with five or more errors.	
Introduction to Patient	Student appropriately introduced self to the patient with one or less errors.	Student appropriately introduced self to the patient with two errors.	Student appropriately introduced self to the patient with three to four errors.	Student failed to appropriately introduce self to the patient or did so with five or more errors.	
Obtained Intake Information	Student appropriately obtained patient intake information with one or less errors.	Student appropriately obtained patient intake information with two errors.	Student appropriately obtained patient intake information with three to four errors.	Student failed to appropriately obtain patient intake information or did so with five or more errors.	
Explanation of Procedure(s)	Student appropriately explained the procedure(s) to the patient with one or less errors.	Student appropriately explained the procedure(s) to the patient with two errors.	Student appropriately explained the procedure(s) to the patient with three to four errors.	Student failed to appropriately explain the procedure(s) to the patient or did so with five or more errors.	
Patient Assessment • **Height** • **Weight** • **Temperature** • **Pulse** • **Respiration** • **Blood Pressure**	Student performed a full patient assessment with two to three errors or omitted one skill assessment.	Student performed a full patient assessment with four to five errors or omitted two skill assessments.	Student performed a full patient assessment with six or more errors or omitted three or more skill assessments.	Student performed a full patient assessment with one to two errors.	
Response to Question 8	Student appropriately responded to the question.	N/A	N/A	Student failed to appropriately respond to the question.	
Response to Question 9	Student appropriately responded to the question.	N/A	N/A	Student failed to appropriately respond to the question.	
Patient Instructions for Hypertension	Student provided appropriate patient instruction with one or less errors.	Student provided appropriate patient instruction with two errors.	Student provided appropriate patient instruction with three to four errors.	Student failed to provide appropriate patient instruction or did so with five or more errors.	

231

Patient Instructions for Weight Loss	Student provided appropriate patient instruction with one or less errors.	Student provided appropriate patient instruction with two errors.	Student provided appropriate patient instruction with three to four errors.	Student failed to provide appropriate patient instruction or did so with five or more errors.
Patient Instructions for Smoking Cessation	Student provided appropriate patient instruction with one or less errors.	Student provided appropriate patient instruction with two errors.	Student provided appropriate patient instruction with three to four errors.	Student failed to provide appropriate patient instruction or did so with five or more errors.
Discussion with Dr. Greggs	Student appropriately discussed the four types of hypertension and their specific characteristics with the physician with one or less errors.	Student appropriately discussed the four types of hypertension and their specific characteristics with the physician with two errors.	Student appropriately discussed the four types of hypertension and their specific characteristics with the physician with three to four errors.	Student failed to appropriately discuss the four types of hypertension and their specific characteristics with the physician or did so with five or more errors.
Documentation	Student properly documented all procedures with one or less errors.	Student properly documented all procedures with two errors or omitted documentation of one procedure.	Student properly documented all procedures with three to four errors or omitted documentation of two procedures.	Student properly documented all procedures with five or more errors or omitted documentation of three or more procedures.
				TOTAL

Based on the above criteria the student's grade for this assignment is: _____

(Total the points for each element scored and average for a final grade.)

Comments to the Student:

Instructor Signature: _____   Date: _____

232

Capillary Puncture, Pediatric Patient

Name _____

Date _____

Agitated Patient

Elements	4 Excellent	3 Proficient	2 Adequate	1 Needs Improvement	Points
Medical Asepsis and Standard Precautions	Student correctly performed medical aseptic techniques and observed all required standard precautions with one or less errors.	Student correctly performed medical aseptic techniques and observed all required standard precautions with two errors.	Student correctly performed medical aseptic techniques and observed all required standard precautions with three to four errors.	Student failed to correctly perform medical aseptic techniques and observe all standard precautions or did so with five or more errors.	
Supplies and Equipment	Student obtained and had available appropriate supplies and equipment with one or less errors.	Student obtained and had available appropriate supplies and equipment with two errors.	Student obtained and had available appropriate supplies and equipment with three to four errors.	Student failed to obtain or have available appropriate supplies and equipment or did so with five or more errors.	
Introduction to Patient	Student appropriately introduced self to the patient with one or less errors.	Student appropriately introduced self to the patient with two errors.	Student appropriately introduced self to the patient with three to four errors.	Student failed to appropriately introduce self to the patient or did so with five or more errors.	
Obtained Intake Information	Student appropriately obtained patient intake information with one or less errors.	Student appropriately obtained patient intake information with two errors.	Student appropriately obtained patient intake information with three to four errors.	Student failed to appropriately obtain patient intake information or did so with five or more errors.	
Establishing a Rapport	Student properly established a rapport with the patient with one or less errors.	Student properly established a rapport with the patient with two errors.	Student properly established a rapport with the patient with three to four errors.	Student failed to properly establish a rapport with the patient or did so with five or more errors.	
Explanation of Procedure(s)	Student appropriately explained the procedure(s) to the patient with one or less errors.	Student appropriately explained the procedure(s) to the patient with two errors.	Student appropriately explained the procedure(s) to the patient with three to four errors.	Student failed to appropriately explain the procedure(s) to the patient or did so with five or more errors.	
Patient Assessment • Height • Weight • Temperature • Pulse • Respiration • Blood Pressure	Student performed a full patient assessment with one to two errors.	Student performed a full patient assessment with two to three errors or omitted one skill assessment.	Student performed a full patient assessment with four to five errors or omitted two skill assessments.	Student performed a full patient assessment with six or more errors or omitted three or more skills.	
STAT order Response to Question 8	Student appropriately answered the question with one or less errors.	Student appropriately answered the question with two errors.	Student appropriately answered the question with three errors.	Student failed to appropriately answer the question or did so with four or more errors.	
Medical Assistant Error Response to Question 9	Student appropriately answered the question with one or less errors.	Student appropriately answered the question with two errors.	Student appropriately answered the question with three errors.	Student failed to appropriately answer the question or did so with four or more errors.	

Elements	4 Excellent	3 Proficient	2 Adequate	1 Needs Improvement	Points
Capillary Puncture	Student properly performed capillary puncture with one or less errors.	Student properly performed capillary puncture with two errors.	Student properly performed capillary puncture with three errors.	Student failed to properly perform capillary puncture or did so with four or more errors.	
Filling Microhematocrit Tubes	Student successfully filled two microhematocrit tubes with one or less errors.	Student successfully filled two microhematocrit tubes with two errors.	Student successfully filled two microhematocrit tubes with three errors or filled one microhematocrit tube.	Student failed to successfully fill two microhematocrit tubes or did so with four or more errors.	
Documentation	Student properly documented all procedures with one or less errors.	Student properly documented all procedures with two errors or omitted documentation of one procedure.	Student properly documented all procedures with three to four errors or omitted documentation of two procedures.	Student properly documented procedures with five or more errors or omitted documentation of three or more procedures.	
				TOTAL	

Nonagitated Patient

Elements	4 Excellent	3 Proficient	2 Adequate	1 Needs Improvement	Points
Medical Asepsis and Standard Precautions	Student correctly performed medical aseptic techniques and observed all required standard precautions with one or less errors.	Student correctly performed medical aseptic techniques and observed all required standard precautions with two errors.	Student correctly performed medical aseptic techniques and observed all required standard precautions with three to four errors.	Student failed to correctly perform medical aseptic techniques and observe all standard precautions or did so with five or more errors.	
Supplies and Equipment	Student obtained and had available appropriate supplies and equipment with one or less errors.	Student obtained and had available appropriate supplies and equipment with two errors.	Student obtained and had available appropriate supplies and equipment with three to four errors.	Student failed to obtain or have available appropriate supplies and equipment or did so with five or more errors.	
Introduction to Patient	Student appropriately introduced self to the patient with one or less errors.	Student appropriately introduced self to the patient with two errors.	Student appropriately introduced self to the patient with three to four errors.	Student failed to appropriately introduce self to the patient or did so with five or more errors.	
Obtained Intake Information	Student appropriately obtained patient intake information with one or less errors.	Student appropriately obtained patient intake information with two errors.	Student appropriately obtained patient intake information with three to four errors.	Student failed to appropriately obtain patient intake information or did so with five or more errors.	
Establishing a Rapport	Student properly established a rapport with the patient with one or less errors.	Student properly established a rapport with the patient with two errors.	Student properly established a rapport with the patient with three to four errors.	Student failed to properly establish a rapport with the patient or did so with five or more errors.	

				Score
Explanation of Procedure(s)	Student appropriately explained the procedure(s) to the patient with one or less errors.	Student appropriately explained the procedure(s) to the patient with two errors.	Student appropriately explained the procedure(s) to the patient with three to four errors.	Student failed to appropriately explain the procedure(s) to the patient or did so with five or more errors.	
Patient Assessment • **Height** • **Weight** • **Temperature** • **Pulse** • **Respiration** • **Blood Pressure**	Student performed a full patient assessment with one to two errors.	Student performed a full patient assessment with two to three errors or omitted one skill assessment.	Student performed a full patient assessment with four to five errors or omitted two skill assessments.	Student performed a full patient assessment with six or more errors or omitted three or more skills.	
STAT order Response to Question 8	Student appropriately answered the question with one or less errors.	Student appropriately answered the question with two errors.	Student appropriately answered the question with three errors.	Student failed to appropriately answer the question or did so with four or more errors.	
Medical Assistant Error Response to Question 9	Student appropriately answered the question with one or less errors.	Student appropriately answered the question with two errors.	Student appropriately answered the question with three errors.	Student failed to appropriately answer the question or did so with four or more errors.	
Capillary Puncture	Student properly performed capillary puncture with one or less errors.	Student properly performed capillary puncture with two errors.	Student properly performed capillary puncture with three errors.	Student failed to properly perform capillary puncture or did so with four or more errors.	
Filling Microhematocrit Tubes	Student successfully filled two microhematocrit tubes with one or less errors.	Student successfully filled two microhematocrit tubes with two errors.	Student successfully filled two microhematocrit tubes with three errors or filled one microhematocrit tube.	Student failed to successfully fill two microhematocrit tubes or did so with four or more errors.	
Documentation	Student properly documented all procedures with one or less errors.	Student properly documented all procedures with two errors or omitted documentation of one procedure.	Student properly documented all procedures with three to four errors or omitted documentation of two procedures.	Student properly documented all procedures with five or more errors or documentation of three or more procedures.	
				TOTAL	

Based on the above criteria the student's grade for this assignment is: _____

(Total the points for each element scored and average for a final grade.)

Comments to the Student:

Instructor Signature: _____   Date: _____

Hypertension–Patient Assessment (Part 1)

Name _____ Date _____

Elements	4 Excellent	3 Proficient	2 Adequate	1 Needs Improvement	Points
Medical Asepsis and Standard Precautions	Student correctly performed medical aseptic techniques and observed all required standard precautions with one or less errors.	Student correctly performed medical aseptic techniques and observed all required standard precautions with two errors.	Student correctly performed medical aseptic techniques and observed all required standard precautions with three to four errors.	Student failed to correctly perform medical aseptic techniques and observe all required standard precautions or did so with five or more errors.	
Supplies and Equipment	Student obtained and had available appropriate supplies and equipment with one or less errors.	Student obtained and had available appropriate supplies and equipment with two errors.	Student obtained and had available appropriate supplies and equipment with three to four errors.	Student failed to obtain or have available appropriate supplies and equipment or did so with five or more errors.	
Introduction to Patient	Student appropriately introduced self to the patient with one or less errors.	Student appropriately introduced self to the patient with two errors.	Student appropriately introduced self to the patient with three to four errors.	Student failed to appropriately introduce self to the patient or did so with five or more errors.	
Obtained Intake Information	Student appropriately obtained patient intake information with one or less errors.	Student appropriately obtained patient intake information with two errors.	Student appropriately obtained patient intake information with three to four errors.	Student failed to appropriately obtain patient intake information or did so with five or more errors.	
Explanation of Procedure(s)	Student appropriately explained the procedure(s) to the patient with one or less errors.	Student appropriately explained the procedure(s) to the patient with two errors.	Student appropriately explained the procedure(s) to the patient with three to four errors.	Student failed to appropriately explain the procedure(s) to the patient or did so with five or more errors.	
Patient Assessment • **Height** • **Weight** • **Temperature** • **Pulse** • **Respiration** • **Blood Pressure**	Student performed a full patient assessment with one to two errors.	Student performed a full patient assessment with two to three errors or omitted one skill assessment.	Student performed a full patient assessment with four to five errors or omitted two skill assessments.	Student performed a full patient assessment with six or more errors or omitted three or more skills.	
Patient Instructions	Student provided appropriate patient instructions with one or less errors.	Student provided patient instructions with two errors.	Student provided patient instructions with three to four errors.	Student failed to provide patient instructions or did so with five or more errors.	
Response to Question 9	Student responded appropriately to question 9 with one or less errors.	Student responded appropriately to question 9 with two errors.	Student responded appropriately to question 9 with three to four errors.	Student failed to respond appropriately to question 9 or did so with five or more errors.	

Course of Action Suggestions	Student provided appropriate course of action suggestion and followed through with a suggestion for a second course of action with one or less errors.	Student provided an acceptable course of action suggestion and followed through with an acceptable suggestion for a second course of action with two errors or provided appropriate course of action suggestion with one or less errors but did not provide a second course of action.	Student provided a course of action suggestion and followed through with a suggestion for a second course of action with three to four errors or provided appropriate course of action suggestion with two errors but did not provide a second course of action.	Student failed to provide an acceptable course of action.
Documentation	Student properly documented all procedures with one or less errors.	Student documented all procedures with two errors or omitted documentation of one procedure.	Student documented all procedures with three to four errors or omitted documentation of two procedures.	Student documented all procedures with five or more errors or omitted documentation of three or more procedures.
				TOTAL

Based on the above criteria the student's grade for this assignment is: _____

(Total the points for each element scored and average for a final grade.)

Comments to the Student:

Instructor Signature: _____   Date: _____

CASE STUDY 37   *Principles of Infection Control*

Name _____   Date _____

Elements	4 Excellent	3 Proficient	2 Adequate	1 Needs Improvement	Points
Role-Play Scenario 1	Student participated in the role-play.	N/A	N/A	Student failed to participate in the role-play.	
Explanation of Instrument Pack Storage	Student accurately explained how long an instrument pack may be stored for it to be considered sterile with no errors.	Student accurately explained how long an instrument pack may be stored for it to be considered sterile with one error.	Student accurately explained how long an instrument pack may be stored for it to be considered sterile with two errors.	Student failed to accurately explain how long an instrument pack may be stored for it to be considered sterile or did so with three or more errors.	
Explanation of Sterilization Process	Student accurately explained the sterilization process with one or less errors.	Student accurately explained the sterilization process with two errors.	Student accurately explained the sterilization process with three errors.	Student failed to accurately explain the sterilization process or did so with four or more errors.	
Inventory	Student accurately performed an inventory of the instruments and instrument packs with one or less errors.	Student accurately performed an inventory of the instruments and instrument packs with two errors.	Student accurately performed an inventory of the instruments and instrument packs with three errors.	Student failed to accurately perform an inventory of the instruments and instrument packs or did so with four or more errors.	
Medical Asepsis and Standard Precautions	Student correctly performed medical aseptic techniques and observed all required standard precautions with one or less errors.	Student correctly performed medical aseptic techniques and observed all required standard precautions with two errors.	Student correctly performed medical aseptic techniques and observed all required standard precautions with three to four errors.	Student failed to correctly perform medical aseptic techniques and observe all required standard precautions or did so with five or more errors.	
Unwrap Instrument Packs	Student unwrapped the instrument packs and appropriately disposed of any disposables contained within the packs.	N/A	N/A	Student failed to unwrap the instrument packs and/or dispose of disposables contained within the pack.	
Sanitization and Disinfection of Instruments	Student accurately sanitized and disinfected the instruments with one or less errors.	Student accurately sanitized and disinfected the instruments with two errors.	Student accurately sanitized and disinfected the instruments with three errors.	Student failed to accurately sanitize and disinfect the instruments or did so with four or more errors.	
Indicator Strip	Student inserted an indicator strip in both packs to be sterilized.	N/A	Student inserted an indicator strip in only one pack.	Student failed to include an indicator strip in the packs to be sterilized.	
Wrapping Instruments	Student used two wraps when preparing the instrument packs for sterilization.	N/A	N/A	Student failed to use two wraps when preparing the instrument packs for sterilization.	

239

Criteria				
Tape Placement and Labeling	Student appropriately placed and labeled the tape before sterilization with no errors.	N/A	N/A	Student failed to appropriately place and label the tape before sterilization or did so with errors.
Instrument Packs • **Small Stack of 2 × 2 Gauze Squares** • **Scalpel Handle** • **Two Hemostats** • **Thumb Tissue Forceps** • **Operating Scissors** • **Needle Holder**	Student included the appropriate items in the instrument packs with no errors.	Student omitted one of the necessary items when preparing the instrument packs.	Student omitted two of the necessary items when preparing the instrument packs.	Student failed to construct the instrument wraps or omitted three or more necessary items when preparing the instrument packs.
Individual Sterilizing Packages	Student prepared individual sterilizing packages for the cervical tenaculum and the curette with one or less errors.	Student prepared individual sterilizing packages for the cervical tenaculum and the curette with two errors.	Student prepared individual sterilizing packages for the cervical tenaculum and the curette with three errors.	Student failed to prepare individual sterilizing packages for the cervical tenaculum and the curette or only prepared one instrument in an individual sterilizing package or prepared both with four or more errors.
Autoclave Sterilization	Student autoclaved the surgical and instrument packs with no errors.	Student autoclaved the surgical and instrument packs with one error.	Student autoclaved the surgical and instrument packs with two errors.	Student failed to autoclave the surgical and instrument packs or failed to autoclave all of it or autoclaved them with three or more errors.
Surgical Packs	Student submitted two surgical packs that contained no errors.	Student submitted two surgical packs that contained one error.	Student submitted two surgical packs that contained two errors.	Student failed to submit two surgical packs or did so and that contained three or more errors.
				TOTAL

Based on the above criteria the student's grade for this assignment is: _____
(Total the points for each element scored and average for a final grade.)

Comments to the Student:

Instructor Signature: _____   Date: _____

CASE STUDY 38   *Well-Baby Check, Pediatrics*

Name _____   Date _____

Elements	4 Excellent	3 Proficient	2 Adequate	1 Needs Improvement	Points
New Patient Chart	Student correctly created a new patient chart electronically and identified the forms required to complete a new patient paper chart with one or less errors.	Student correctly created a new patient chart electronically and identified the forms required to complete a new patient paper chart with two errors.	Student correctly created a new patient chart electronically and identified the forms required to complete a new patient paper chart with three to four errors.	Student failed to correctly create a new patient chart electronically and identify the forms required to complete a new patient paper chart or did so with five or more errors.	
Supplies and Equipment	Student obtained and had available appropriate supplies and equipment with one or less errors.	Student obtained and had available appropriate supplies and equipment with two errors.	Student obtained and had available appropriate supplies and equipment with three to four errors.	Student failed to obtain or have available appropriate supplies and equipment or did so with five or more errors.	
Medical Asepsis and Standard Precautions	Student correctly performed medical aseptic techniques and observed all required standard precautions with one or less errors.	Student correctly performed medical aseptic techniques and observed all required standard precautions with two errors.	Student correctly performed medical aseptic techniques and observed all required standard precautions with three to four errors.	Student failed to correctly perform medical aseptic techniques and observe all required standard precautions or did so with five or more errors.	
Introduction to Patient and Patient's Mother	Student appropriately introduced self to the patient and patient's mother with one or less errors.	Student appropriately introduced self to the patient and patient's mother with two errors.	Student appropriately introduced self to the patient and patient's mother with three to four errors.	Student failed to appropriately introduce self to the patient and patient's mother or did so with five or more errors.	
Obtained Intake Information	Student appropriately obtained patient intake information with one or less errors.	Student appropriately obtained patient intake information with two errors.	Student appropriately obtained patient intake information with three to four errors.	Student failed to appropriately obtain patient intake information or did so with five or more errors.	
Obtained Consent	Student appropriately obtained employee consent with one or less errors.	Student appropriately obtained employee consent with two errors.	Student appropriately obtained employee consent with three to four errors.	Student failed to appropriately obtain employee consent or did so with five or more errors.	
Patient Assessment • Length • Weight • Temperature • Head Circumference	Student performed a full patient assessment with one to two errors.	Student performed a full patient assessment with two to three errors or omitted one skill assessment.	Student performed a full patient assessment with four to five errors or omitted two skill assessments.	Student performed a full patient assessment with six or more errors or omitted three or more skills.	

241

	Student provided the physician with the appropriate supplies and equipment with one or less errors.	Student provided the physician with the appropriate supplies and equipment with two errors.	Student provided the physician with the appropriate supplies and equipment with three to four errors.	Student failed to provide the physician with the appropriate supplies and equipment or did so with six or more errors.	
Supplies and Equipment Identified for the Physical Examination					
Growth Chart	Student properly documented length, weight, and head circumference on an appropriate growth chart with one or less errors.	Student properly documented length, weight, and head circumference on an appropriate growth chart with two errors.	Student properly documented length, weight, and head circumference on an appropriate growth chart with three errors.	Student failed to properly document length, weight, and head circumference on an appropriate growth chart or did so with four or more errors.	
Documentation	Student properly documented all procedures with one or less errors.	Student properly documented all procedures with two errors or omitted documentation of one procedure.	Student properly documented all procedures with three to four errors or omitted documentation of two procedures.	Student properly documented all procedures with five or more errors or omitted documentation of three or more procedures.	
				TOTAL	

Based on the above criteria the student's grade for this assignment is: _____

(Total the points for each element scored and average for a final grade.)

Comments to the Student:

Instructor Signature: _____   Date: _____

Hypertension–Patient Assessment (Part 2)

Name _____ Date _____

Elements	4 Excellent	3 Proficient	2 Adequate	1 Needs Improvement	Points
Medical Asepsis and Standard Precautions	Student correctly performed medical aseptic techniques and observed all required standard precautions with one or less errors.	Student correctly performed medical aseptic techniques and observed all required standard precautions with two errors.	Student correctly performed medical aseptic techniques and observed all required standard precautions with three to four errors.	Student failed to correctly perform medical aseptic techniques and observe all required standard precautions or did so with five or more errors.	
Supplies and Equipment	Student obtained and had available appropriate supplies and equipment with one or less errors.	Student obtained and had available appropriate supplies and equipment with two errors.	Student obtained and had available appropriate supplies and equipment with three to four errors.	Student failed to obtain or have available appropriate supplies and equipment or did so with five or more errors.	
Introduction to Patient	Student appropriately introduced self to the patient with one or less errors.	Student appropriately introduced self to the patient with two errors.	Student appropriately introduced self to the patient with three to four errors.	Student failed to appropriately introduce self to the patient or did so with five or more errors.	
Obtained Intake Information	Student appropriately obtained patient intake information with one or less errors.	Student appropriately obtained patient intake information with two errors.	Student appropriately obtained patient intake information with three to four errors.	Student failed to appropriately obtain patient intake information or did so with five or more errors.	
Explanation of Procedure(s)	Student provided appropriate explanation of procedure(s) with one or less errors.	Student provided appropriate explanation of procedure(s) with two errors.	Student provided appropriate explanation of procedure(s) with three to four errors.	Student failed to provide appropriate explanation of procedure(s) or did so with five or more errors.	
Patient Assessment MONDAY • **Height** • **Weight** • **Temperature** • **Pulse** • **Respiration** • **Blood Pressure**	Student performed a full patient assessment with one to two errors.	Student performed a full patient assessment with two to three errors or omitted one skill assessment.	Student performed a full patient assessment with four to five errors or omitted two skill assessments.	Student performed a full patient assessment with six or more errors or omitted three or more skills.	
Patient Assessment WEDNESDAY • **Height** • **Weight** • **Temperature** • **Pulse** • **Respiration** • **Blood Pressure**	Student performed a full patient assessment with one to two errors.	Student performed a full patient assessment with two to three errors or omitted one skill assessment.	Student performed a full patient assessment with four to five errors or omitted two skill assessments.	Student performed a full patient assessment with six or more errors or omitted three or more skills.	

Patient Assessment FRIDAY • Height • Weight • Temperature • Pulse • Respiration • Blood Pressure	Student performed a full patient assessment with one to two errors.	Student performed a full patient assessment with two to three errors or omitted one skill assessment.	Student performed a full patient assessment with four to five errors or omitted two skill assessments.	Student performed a full patient assessment with six or more errors or omitted three or more skills.	
Patient Instructions	Student provided appropriate patient instruction with one or less errors.	Student provided appropriate patient instruction with two errors.	Student provided appropriate patient instruction with three to four errors.	Student failed to provide appropriate patient instructions or did so with five or more errors.	
Conversation with Dr. Wertz	Student reported results and medication compliance appropriately with one or less errors.	Student reported results and medication compliance appropriately with two to three errors.	Student reported results and medication compliance appropriately with four to five errors.	Student failed to appropriately report results and medication compliance or did so with six or more errors.	
Documentation	Student properly documented all procedures with one or less errors.	Student properly documented all procedures with two errors or omitted documentation of one procedure.	Student properly documented all procedures with three to four errors or omitted documentation of two procedures.	Student properly documented all procedures with five or more errors or omitted documentation of three or more procedures.	
				TOTAL	

Based on the above criteria the student's grade for this assignment is: _____

(Total the points for each element scored and average for a final grade.)

Comments to the Student:

Instructor Signature: _____   Date: _____

Capillary Puncture, INR Point-of-Care Testing

Name _____

Date _____

Elements	4 Excellent	3 Proficient	2 Adequate	1 Needs Improvement	Points
New Patient Chart	Student correctly created a new patient chart electronically and identified the forms requiring a patient signature with one or less errors.	Student correctly created a new patient chart electronically and identified the forms requiring a patient signature with two errors.	Student correctly created a new patient chart electronically and identified the forms requiring a patient signature with three to four errors.	Student failed to correctly create a new patient chart electronically and identify the forms requiring a patient signature or did so with five or more errors.	
Supplies and Equipment	Student obtained and had available appropriate supplies and equipment with one or less errors.	Student obtained and had available appropriate supplies and equipment with two errors.	Student obtained and had available appropriate supplies and equipment with three to four errors.	Student failed to obtain or have available appropriate supplies and equipment or did so with five or more errors.	
Medical Asepsis and Standard Precautions	Student correctly performed medical aseptic techniques and observed all required standard precautions with one or less errors.	Student correctly performed medical aseptic techniques and observed all required standard precautions with two errors.	Student correctly performed medical aseptic techniques and observed all required standard precautions with three to four errors.	Student failed to correctly perform medical aseptic techniques and observe all required standard precautions or did so with five or more errors.	
Introduction to Patient	Student appropriately introduced self to the patient with one or less errors.	Student appropriately introduced self to the patient with two errors.	Student appropriately introduced self to the patient with three to four errors.	Student failed to appropriately introduce self to the patient or did so with five or more errors.	
Obtained Intake Information	Student appropriately obtained patient intake information with one or less errors.	Student appropriately obtained patient intake information with two errors.	Student appropriately obtained patient intake information with three to four errors.	Student failed to appropriately obtain patient intake information or did so with five or more errors.	
Explanation of Procedure(s)	Student appropriately explained the procedure(s) to the patient with one or less errors.	Student appropriately explained the procedure(s) to the patient with two errors.	Student appropriately explained the procedure(s) to the patient with three to four errors.	Student failed to appropriately explain the procedure(s) to the patient or did so with five or more errors.	
Patient Assessment • Height • Weight • Temperature • Pulse • Respiration • Blood Pressure	Student performed a full patient assessment with one to two errors.	Student performed a full patient assessment with two to three errors or omitted one skill assessment.	Student performed a full patient assessment with four to five errors or omitted two skill assessments.	Student performed a full patient assessment with six or more errors or omitted three or more skills.	

	Student provided appropriate patient instruction with one or less errors.	Student provided appropriate patient instruction with two errors.	Student provided appropriate patient instruction with three to four errors.	Student failed to provide appropriate patient instruction or did so with five or more errors.	
Patient Instructions/ Preparation	Student provided appropriate patient instruction with one or less errors.	Student provided appropriate patient instruction with two errors.	Student provided appropriate patient instruction with three to four errors.	Student failed to provide appropriate patient instruction or did so with five or more errors.	
Patient Capillary Puncture	Student properly performed capillary puncture with one or less errors.	Student properly performed capillary puncture with two errors.	Student properly performed capillary puncture with three errors.	Student failed to properly perform capillary puncture or did so with four or more errors.	
INR Point-of-Care Test	Student successfully completed an INR test with one or less errors.	Student successfully completed an INR test with two errors.	Student successfully completed an INR test with three to four errors.	Student failed to successfully complete an INR test or did so with five or more errors.	
Response to Question 11	Student appropriately responded to the question.	N/A	N/A	Student failed to appropriately respond to the question.	
Documentation	Student properly documented all procedures with one or less errors.	Student properly documented all procedures with two errors or omitted documentation of one procedure.	Student properly documented all procedures with three to four errors or omitted documentation of two procedures.	Student properly documented all procedures with five or more errors or omitted documentation of three or more procedures.	
				TOTAL	

Based on the above criteria the student's grade for this assignment is: _____

(Total the points for each element scored and average for a final grade.)

Comments to the Student:

Instructor Signature: _____ Date: _____

CASE STUDY 41 *Pap Smear and Breast Examination*

Name _____ Date _____

Elements	4 Excellent	3 Proficient	2 Adequate	1 Needs Improvement	Points
Appointment Scheduling	Student correctly scheduled an appointment and obtained the required information with one or less errors.	Students correctly scheduled an appointment and obtained the required information with two errors.	Student correctly scheduled an appointment and obtained the required information with three to four errors.	Student failed to correctly schedule an appointment and/or failed to obtain the required information or did so with five or more errors.	
Supplies and Equipment	Student obtained and had available appropriate supplies and equipment with one or less errors.	Student obtained and had available appropriate supplies and equipment with two errors.	Student obtained and had available appropriate supplies and equipment with three to four errors.	Student failed to obtain or have available appropriate supplies and equipment or did so with five or more errors.	
Patient Instructions via Telephone	Student provided appropriate patient instructions with one or less errors.	Student provided appropriate patient instructions with two errors.	Student provided appropriate patient instructions with three to four errors.	Student failed to provide appropriate patient instructions or did so with five or more errors.	
Telephone Etiquette	Student correctly applied proper telephone etiquette with one or less errors.	Student correctly applied proper telephone etiquette with two errors.	Student correctly applied proper telephone etiquette with three to four errors.	Student failed to correctly apply proper telephone etiquette or did so with five or more errors.	
New Patient Chart	Student correctly assembled a new patient chart and completed all forms with one or less errors.	Student correctly assembled a new patient chart and completed all forms with two errors.	Student correctly assembled a new patient chart and completed all forms with three to four errors.	Student failed to correctly assemble a new patient chart and/or failed to complete all forms or did so with five or more errors.	
Medical Asepsis and Standard Precautions	Student correctly performed medical aseptic techniques and observed all required standard precautions with one or less errors.	Student correctly performed medical aseptic techniques and observed all required standard precautions with two errors.	Student correctly performed medical aseptic techniques and observed all required standard precautions with three to four errors.	Student failed to correctly perform medical aseptic techniques and observe all required standard precautions or did so with five or more errors.	
Response to Question 7	Student responded appropriately to question 7 with one or less errors.	Student responded appropriately to question 7 with two errors.	Student responded appropriately to question 7 with three to four errors.	Student failed to respond appropriately to question 7 or did so with five or more errors.	
Introduction to Patient	Student appropriately introduced self to the patient with one or less errors.	Student appropriately introduced self to the patient with two errors.	Student appropriately introduced self to the patient with three to four errors.	Student failed to appropriately introduce self to the patient or did so with five or more errors.	

Criteria	1	2	3	4
Obtained Intake Information	Student appropriately obtained patient intake information with one or less errors.	Student appropriately obtained patient intake information with two errors.	Student appropriately obtained patient intake information with three to four errors.	Student failed to appropriately obtain patient intake information or did so with five or more errors.
Response to Question 11	Student responded appropriately to question 11 with one or less errors.	Student responded appropriately to question 11 with two errors.	Student responded appropriately to question 11 with three to four errors.	Student failed to respond appropriately to question 11 or did so with five or more errors.
Obtained Consent	Student appropriately obtained patient consent with one or less errors.	Student appropriately obtained patient consent with two errors.	Student appropriately obtained patient consent with three to four errors.	Student failed to appropriately obtain patient consent or did so with five or more errors.
Patient Assessment	Student performed a full patient assessment with one to two errors.	Student performed a full patient assessment with two to three errors or omitted one skill assessment.	Student performed a full patient assessment with four to five errors or omitted two skill assessments.	Student performed a full patient assessment with six or more errors or omitted three or more skills.
Explanation of Disrobing, Gowning, and Draping	Student appropriately explained how to disrobe, gown, and drape for the procedures with one or less errors.	Student appropriately explained how to disrobe, gown, and drape for the procedures with two errors.	Student appropriately explained how to disrobe, gown, and drape for the procedures with three to four errors.	Student failed to appropriately explain how to disrobe, gown, and drape for the procedures or did so with five or more errors.
Explanation of Procedure(s)	Student appropriately explained the procedure(s) to the patient with one or less errors.	Student appropriately explained the procedure(s) to the patient with two errors.	Student appropriately explained the procedure(s) to the patient with three to four errors.	Student failed to appropriately explain the procedure(s) to the patient or did so with five or more errors.
Patient Positioning	Student appropriately positioned and draped the patient for all three procedures with one or less errors.	Student appropriately positioned and draped the patient for all three procedures with two errors.	Student appropriately positioned and draped the patient for all three procedures with three to four errors.	Student failed to appropriately position and drape the patient for all three procedures or did so with five or more errors.
Assisting the Physician in Pelvic Examination	Student appropriately assisted the physician as required with one or less errors.	Student appropriately assisted the physician as required with two errors.	Student appropriately assisted the physician as required with three to four errors.	Student appropriately assisted the physician as required or did so with five or more errors.
Assisting the Physician in Pap Smear	Student appropriately assisted the physician as required with one or less errors.	Student appropriately assisted the physician as required with two errors.	Student appropriately assisted the physician as required with three to four errors.	Student appropriately assisted the physician as required or did so with five or more errors.
Assisting the Physician in Breast Examination	Student appropriately assisted the physician as required with one or less errors.	Student appropriately assisted the physician as required with two errors.	Student appropriately assisted the physician as required with three to four errors.	Student appropriately assisted the physician as required or did so with five or more errors.

	Student appropriately labeled the slide/vial for transport to the laboratory with one or less errors.	Student appropriately labeled the slide/vial for transport to the laboratory with two errors.	Student appropriately labeled the slide/vial for transport to the laboratory with three to four hours.	Student failed to appropriately label the slide/vial for transport to the laboratory or did so with five or more errors.	
Preparation of Slide/Vial for Transport to Laboratory					
Documentation	Student properly documented all procedures with one or less errors.	Student properly documented all procedures with two errors or omitted documentation of one procedure.	Student properly documented all procedures with three to four errors or omitted documentation of two procedures.	Student properly documented all procedures with five or more errors or omitted documentation of three or more procedures.	
					TOTAL

Based on the above criteria the student's grade for this assignment is: _____

(Total the points for each element scored and average for a final grade.)

Comments to the Student:

Instructor Signature: _____ Date: _____

CASE STUDY 42 *Preoperative Examination and Laboratory Tests*

Elements	4 Excellent	3 Proficient	2 Adequate	1 Needs Improvement	Points
Medical Asepsis and Standard Precautions	Student correctly performed medical aseptic techniques and observed all required standard precautions with one or less errors.	Student correctly performed medical aseptic techniques and observed all required standard precautions with two errors.	Student correctly performed medical aseptic techniques and observed all required standard precautions with three to four errors.	Student failed to correctly perform medical aseptic techniques and observe all required standard precautions or did so with five or more errors.	
Supplies and Equipment	Student obtained and had available appropriate supplies and equipment with one or less errors.	Student obtained and had available appropriate supplies and equipment with two errors.	Student obtained and had available appropriate supplies and equipment with three to four errors.	Student failed to obtain or have available appropriate supplies and equipment or did so with five or more errors.	
Introduction to Patient	Student appropriately introduced self to the patient with one or less errors.	Student appropriately introduced self to the patient with two errors.	Student appropriately introduced self to the patient with three to four errors.	Student failed to appropriately introduce self to the patient or did so with five or more errors.	
Obtained Intake Information	Student appropriately obtained patient intake information with one or less errors.	Student appropriately obtained patient intake information with two errors.	Student appropriately obtained patient intake information with three to four errors.	Student failed to appropriately obtain patient intake information or did so with five or more errors.	
Explanation of Procedure(s)	Student appropriately explained the procedure(s) to the patient with one or less errors.	Student appropriately explained the procedure(s) to the patient with two errors.	Student appropriately explained the procedure(s) to the patient with three to four errors.	Student failed to appropriately explain the procedure(s) to the patient or did so with five or more errors.	
Obtained Consent	Student appropriately obtained patient consent with one or less errors.	Student appropriately obtained patient consent with two errors.	Student appropriately obtained patient consent with three to four errors.	Student failed to appropriately obtain patient consent or did so with five or more errors.	
Patient Assessment • Height • Weight • Temperature • Pulse • Respiration • Blood Pressure	Student performed a full patient assessment with one to two errors.	Student performed a full patient assessment with two to three errors or omitted one skill assessment.	Student performed a full patient assessment with four to five errors or omitted two skill assessments.	Student performed a full patient assessment with six or more errors or omitted three or more skills.	
Patient Instructions	Student provided appropriate patient instructions with one or less errors.	Student provided appropriate patient instructions with two errors.	Student provided appropriate patient instructions with three to four errors.	Student failed to provide appropriate patient instructions or did so with five or more errors.	

	Student properly performed a venipuncture with one or less errors.	Student properly performed a venipuncture with two errors.	Student properly performed a venipuncture with three to four errors.	Student failed to properly perform a venipuncture or did so with five or more errors.	
Perform Venipuncture					
Correct Number and Color-Topped Tubes	Student obtained blood in the correct number and color-topped tubes with one or less errors.	Student obtained blood in the correct number and color-topped tubes with two errors.	Student obtained blood in the correct number and color-topped tubes with three to four errors.	Student failed to obtain blood in the correct number and color-topped tubes or did so with five or more errors.	
Response to Question 11	Student responded appropriately to question 11 with one or less errors.	Student responded appropriately to question 11 with two errors.	Student responded appropriately to question 11 with three to four errors.	Student failed to respond appropriately to question 11 or did so with five or more errors.	
Package Specimens for Laboratory	Student properly packaged the specimens to be sent to the laboratory with one or less errors.	Student properly packaged the specimens to be sent to the laboratory with two errors.	Student properly packaged the specimens to be sent to the laboratory with three to four errors.	Student failed to properly package the specimens to be sent to the laboratory or did so with five or more errors.	
Schedule Chest X-ray, Operating Room, and Hospital Stay	Student properly scheduled chest X-ray, operating room, and hospital stay with one or less errors.	Student properly scheduled chest X-ray, operating room, and hospital stay with two errors.	Student properly scheduled chest X-ray, operating room, and hospital stay with three to four errors.	Student failed to properly schedule chest X-ray, operating room, and hospital stay or did so with five or more errors.	
Response to Question 14	Student responded appropriately to question 14 with one or less errors.	Student responded appropriately to question 14 with two errors.	Student responded appropriately to question 14 with three to four errors.	Student failed to respond appropriately to question 14 or did so with five or more errors.	
Documentation	Student properly documented all procedures with one or less errors.	Student properly documented all procedures with two errors or omitted documentation of one procedure.	Student properly documented all procedures with three to four errors or omitted documentation of two procedures.	Student properly documented all procedures with five or more errors or omitted documentation of three or more procedures.	
				TOTAL	

Based on the above criteria the student's grade for this assignment is: _____

(Total the points for each element scored and average for a final grade.)

Comments to the Student:

Instructor Signature: _____ Date: _____

CASE STUDY 43 *Vaccinations, Influenza*

Name _____ Date _____

Employee 1

Elements	4 Excellent	3 Proficient	2 Adequate	1 Needs Improvement	Points
Medical Asepsis and Standard Precautions	Student correctly performed medical aseptic techniques and observed all required standard precautions with one or less errors.	Student correctly performed medical aseptic techniques and observed all required standard precautions with two errors.	Student correctly performed medical aseptic techniques and observed all required standard precautions with three to four errors.	Student failed to correctly perform medical aseptic techniques and observe all required standard precautions or did so with five or more errors.	
Supplies and Equipment	Student obtained and had available appropriate supplies and equipment with one or less errors.	Student obtained and had available appropriate supplies and equipment with two errors.	Student obtained and had available appropriate supplies and equipment with three to four errors.	Student failed to obtain or have available appropriate supplies and equipment or did so with five or more errors.	
Introduction to Employee	Student appropriately introduced self to the employee with one or less errors.	Student appropriately introduced self to the employee with two errors.	Student appropriately introduced self to the employee with three to four errors.	Student failed to appropriately introduce self to the employee or did so with five or more errors.	
Obtained Intake Information	Student appropriately obtained employee intake information with one or less errors.	Student appropriately obtained employee intake information with two errors.	Student appropriately obtained employee intake information with three to four errors.	Student failed to appropriately obtain employee intake information or did so with five or more errors.	
Explanation of Procedure(s)	Student appropriately explained the procedure(s) to the employee including risks and side effects with one or less errors.	Student appropriately explained the procedure(s) to the employee including risks and side effects with two errors.	Student appropriately explained the procedure(s) to the employee including risks and side effects with three to four errors.	Student failed to appropriately explain the procedure(s) to the employee including risks and side effects or did so with five or more errors.	
Obtained Consent	Student appropriately obtained employee consent with one or less errors.	Student appropriately obtained employee consent with two errors.	Student appropriately obtained employee consent with three to four errors.	Student failed to appropriately obtain employee consent or did so with five or more errors.	
Patient Assessment • Height • Weight • Temperature • Pulse • Respiration • Blood Pressure	Student performed a full patient assessment with one to two errors.	Student performed a full patient assessment with two to three errors or omitted one skill assessment.	Student performed a full patient assessment with four to five errors or omitted two skill assessments.	Student performed a full patient assessment with six or more errors or omitted three or more skills.	

	4 Excellent	3 Proficient	2 Adequate	1 Needs Improvement	Points
Subcutaneous Injection	Student properly performed a subcutaneous injection with one or less errors.	Student properly performed a subcutaneous injection with two errors.	Student properly performed a subcutaneous injection with three errors.	Student failed to properly perform a subcutaneous injection or did so with four or more errors.	
Documentation	Student properly documented all procedures with one or less errors.	Student properly documented all procedures with two errors or omitted documentation of one procedure.	Student properly documented all procedures with three to four errors or omitted documentation of two procedures.	Student properly documented all procedures with five or more errors or omitted documentation of three or more procedures.	
				TOTAL	

Employee 2

Elements	4 Excellent	3 Proficient	2 Adequate	1 Needs Improvement	Points
Medical Asepsis and Standard Precautions	Student correctly performed medical aseptic techniques and observed all required standard precautions with one or less errors.	Student correctly performed medical aseptic techniques and observed all required standard precautions with two errors.	Student correctly performed medical aseptic techniques and observed all required standard precautions with three to four errors.	Student failed to correctly perform medical aseptic techniques and observe all required standard precautions or did so with five or more errors.	
Supplies and Equipment	Student obtained and had available appropriate supplies and equipment with one or less errors.	Student obtained and had available appropriate supplies and equipment with two errors.	Student obtained and had available appropriate supplies and equipment with three to four errors.	Student failed to obtain or have available appropriate supplies and equipment or did so with five or more errors.	
Introduction to Employee	Student appropriately introduced self to the employee with one or less errors.	Student appropriately introduced self to the employee with two errors.	Student appropriately introduced self to the employee with three to four errors.	Student failed to appropriately introduce self to the employee or did so with five or more errors.	
Obtained Intake Information	Student appropriately obtained employee intake information with one or less errors.	Student appropriately obtained employee intake information with two errors.	Student appropriately obtained employee intake information with three to four errors.	Student failed to appropriately obtain employee intake information or did so with five or more errors.	
Explanation of Procedure(s)	Student appropriately explained the procedure(s) to the employee including risks and side effects with one or less errors.	Student appropriately explained the procedure(s) to the employee including risks and side effects with two errors.	Student appropriately explained the procedure(s) to the employee including risks and side effects with three to four errors.	Student failed to appropriately explain the procedure(s) to the employee including risks and side effects or did so with five or more errors.	
Obtained Consent	Student appropriately obtained employee consent with one or less errors.	Student appropriately obtained employee consent with two errors.	Student appropriately obtained employee consent with three to four errors.	Student failed to appropriately obtain employee consent or did so with five or more errors.	

Elements	Excellent	Proficient	Adequate	Needs Improvement	Points
Patient Assessment • Height • Weight • Temperature • Pulse • Respiration • Blood pressure	Student performed a full patient assessment with one to two errors.	Student performed a full patient assessment with two to three errors or omitted one skill assessment.	Student performed a full patient assessment with four to five errors or omitted two skill assessments.	Student performed a full patient assessment with six or more errors or omitted three or more skills.	
Subcutaneous Injection	Student properly performed a subcutaneous injection with one or less errors.	Student properly performed a subcutaneous injection with two errors.	Student properly performed a subcutaneous injection with three errors.	Student failed to properly perform a subcutaneous injection or did so with four or more errors.	
Response to Condition Question 11	Student properly assessed and responded to employee condition with one or less errors.	Student properly assessed and responded to employee condition with two errors.	Student properly assessed and responded to employee condition with three to four errors.	Student failed to properly assess or respond to employee condition or did so with five or more errors.	
Documentation	Student properly documented all procedures with one or less errors.	Student properly documented all procedures with two errors or omitted documentation of one procedure.	Student properly documented all procedures with three to four errors or omitted documentation of two procedures.	Student properly documented all procedures with five or more errors or omitted documentation of three or more procedures.	
				TOTAL	

Employee 3

Elements	4 Excellent	3 Proficient	2 Adequate	1 Needs Improvement	Points
Medical Asepsis and Standard Precautions	Student correctly performed medical aseptic techniques and observed all required standard precautions with one or less errors.	Student correctly performed medical aseptic techniques and observed all required standard precautions with two errors.	Student correctly performed medical aseptic techniques and observed all required standard precautions with three to four errors.	Student failed to correctly perform medical aseptic techniques and observe all required standard precautions or did so with five or more errors.	
Supplies and Equipment	Student obtained and had available appropriate supplies and equipment with one or less errors.	Student obtained and had available appropriate supplies and equipment with two errors.	Student obtained and had available appropriate supplies and equipment with three to four errors.	Student failed to obtain or have available appropriate supplies and equipment or did so with five or more errors.	
Introduction to Employee	Student appropriately introduced self to the employee with one or less errors.	Student appropriately introduced self to the employee with two errors.	Student appropriately introduced self to the employee with three to four errors.	Student failed to appropriately introduce self to the employee or did so with five or more errors.	
Obtained Intake Information	Student appropriately obtained employee intake information with one or less errors.	Student appropriately obtained employee intake information with two errors.	Student appropriately obtained employee intake information with three to four errors.	Student failed to appropriately obtain employee intake information or did so with five or more errors.	

Explanation of Procedure(s)	Student appropriately explained the procedure(s) to the employee including risks and side effects with one or less errors.	Student appropriately explained the procedure(s) to the employee including risks and side effects with two errors.	Student appropriately explained the procedure(s) to the employee including risks and side effects with three to four errors.	Student failed to appropriately explain the procedure(s) to the employee including risks and side effects or did so with five or more errors.
Obtained Consent	Student appropriately obtained employee consent with one or less errors.	Student appropriately obtained employee consent with two errors.	Student appropriately obtained employee consent with three to four errors.	Student failed to appropriately obtain employee consent or did so with five or more errors.
Patient Assessment • **Height** • **Weight** • **Temperature** • **Pulse** • **Respiration** • **Blood Pressure**	Student performed a full patient assessment with one to two errors.	Student performed a full patient assessment with two to three errors or omitted one skill assessment.	Student performed a full patient assessment with four to five errors or omitted two skill assessments.	Student performed a full patient assessment with six or more errors or omitted three or more skills.
Subcutaneous Injection	Student properly performed a subcutaneous injection with one or less errors.	Student properly performed a subcutaneous injection with two errors.	Student properly performed a subcutaneous injection with three errors.	Student failed to properly perform a subcutaneous injection or did so with four or more errors.
Documentation	Student properly documented all procedures with one or less errors.	Student properly documented all procedures with two errors or omitted documentation of one procedure.	Student properly documented all procedures with three to four errors or omitted documentation of two procedures.	Student properly documented all procedures with five or more errors or omitted documentation of three or more procedures.
				TOTAL

Based on the above criteria the student's grade for this assignment is: _____

(Total the points for each element scored and average for a final grade.)

Comments to the Student:

Instructor Signature: _____   Date: _____

Digestive Disorder

Name _____ Date _____

Elements	4 Excellent	3 Proficient	2 Adequate	1 Needs Improvement	Points
New Patient Chart	Student correctly assembled a new patient chart and completed all forms with one or less errors.	Student correctly assembled a new patient chart and completed all forms with two errors.	Student correctly assembled a new patient chart and completed all forms with three to four errors.	Student failed to correctly assemble a new patient chart and/or failed to complete all forms or did so with five or more errors.	
Medical Asepsis and Standard Precautions	Student correctly performed medical aseptic techniques and observed all required standard precautions with one or less errors.	Student correctly performed medical aseptic techniques and observed all required standard precautions with two errors.	Student correctly performed medical aseptic techniques and observed all required standard precautions with three to four errors.	Student failed to correctly perform medical aseptic techniques and observe all required standard precautions or did so with five or more errors.	
Supplies and Equipment	Student obtained and had available appropriate supplies and equipment with one or less errors.	Student obtained and had available appropriate supplies and equipment with two errors.	Student obtained and had available appropriate supplies and equipment with three to four errors.	Student failed to obtain or have available appropriate supplies and equipment or did so with five or more errors.	
Introduction to Patient	Student appropriately introduced self to the patient with one or less errors.	Student appropriately introduced self to the patient with two errors.	Student appropriately introduced self to the patient with three to four errors.	Student failed to appropriately introduce self to the patient or did so with five or more errors.	
Obtained Intake Information	Student appropriately obtained patient intake information with one or less errors.	Student appropriately obtained patient intake information with two errors.	Student appropriately obtained patient intake information with three to four errors.	Student failed to appropriately obtain patient intake information or did so with five or more errors.	
Obtained Consent	Student appropriately obtained patient consent with one or less errors.	Student appropriately obtained patient consent with two errors.	Student appropriately obtained patient consent with three to four errors.	Student failed to appropriately obtain patient consent or did so with five or more errors.	
Patient Assessment	Student performed a full patient assessment with one to two errors.	Student performed a full patient assessment with two to three errors or omitted one skill assessment.	Student performed a full patient assessment with four to five errors or omitted two skill assessments.	Student performed a full patient assessment with six or more errors or omitted three or more skills.	
Explanation of Disrobing, Gowning, and Draping	Student appropriately explained how to disrobe, gown, and drape for the procedures with one or less errors.	Student appropriately explained how to disrobe, gown, and drape for the procedures with two errors.	Student appropriately explained how to disrobe, gown, and drape for the procedures with three to four errors.	Student failed to appropriately explain how to disrobe, gown, and drape for the procedures or did so with five or more errors.	
Assisting the Physician with Procedures	Student appropriately assisted the physician as required with one or less errors.	Student appropriately assisted the physician as required with two errors.	Student appropriately assisted the physician as required with three to four errors.	Student failed to appropriately assist the physician as required or did so with five or more errors.	
Perform Venipuncture	Student properly performed a venipuncture with one or less errors.	Student properly performed a venipuncture with two errors.	Student properly performed a venipuncture with three to four errors.	Student failed to properly perform a venipuncture or did so with five or more errors.	

Criteria	Student obtained/performed with one or less errors	Student obtained/performed with two errors	Student obtained/performed with three to four errors	Student failed / five or more errors	Score
Collect Correct Number and Color-Topped Tubes and Identify Correct Order of Draw	Student obtained blood in the correct number and color-topped tubes with one or less errors.	Student obtained blood in the correct number and color-topped tubes with two errors.	Student obtained blood in the correct number and color-topped tubes with three to four errors.	Student failed to obtain blood in the correct number and color-topped tubes or did so with five or more errors.	
Package Specimens for Laboratory (Specimens were properly collected and labeled)	Student properly packaged the specimens to be sent to the laboratory with one or less errors.	Student properly packaged the specimens to be sent to the laboratory with two errors.	Student properly packaged the specimens to be sent to the laboratory with three to four errors.	Student failed to properly package the specimens to be sent to the laboratory or did so with five or more errors.	
Perform CBC	Student properly performed a CBC with one or less errors.	Student properly performed a CBC with two errors.	Student properly performed a CBC with three to four errors.	Student failed to properly perform a CBC or did so with five or more errors.	
Explanation of Sigmoidoscopy Procedure	Student appropriately explained the procedure to the patient with one or less errors.	Student appropriately explained the procedure to the patient with two errors.	Student appropriately explained the procedure to the patient with three to four errors.	Student failed to appropriately explain the procedure to the patient or did so with five or more errors.	
Schedule and Provide Patient with Procedure Time	Student appropriately performed these tasks with one or less errors.	Student appropriately performed these tasks with two errors.	Student appropriately performed these tasks with three errors.	Student failed to perform these tasks or did so with four or more errors.	
Explanation for Obtaining Stool Sample	Student appropriately explained the procedure to the patient with one or less errors.	Student appropriately explained the procedure to the patient with two errors.	Student appropriately explained the procedure to the patient with three to four errors.	Student failed to appropriately explain the procedure to the patient or did so with five or more errors.	
Response in Writing to Question 14 (a-g)	Student responded appropriately to question 14 (a-g) with one or less errors.	Student responded appropriately to question 14 (a-g) with two errors.	Student responded appropriately to question 14 (a-g) or did so with three to four errors.	Student failed to respond appropriately to question 14 (a-g) or did so with five or more errors.	
Documentation	Student properly documented all procedures with one or less errors.	Student properly documented all procedures with two errors or omitted documentation of one procedure.	Student properly documented all procedures with three to four errors or omitted documentation of two procedures.	Student properly documented all procedures with five or more errors or omitted documentation of three or more procedures.	
				TOTAL	

Based on the above criteria the student's grade for this assignment is: _____

(Total the points for each element scored and average for a final grade.)

Comments to the Student:

Instructor Signature: _____   Date: _____

Physical Examination, Immunizations, and PPD

Name _____

Date _____

Elements	4 Excellent	3 Proficient	2 Adequate	1 Needs Improvement	Points
New Patient Chart	Student correctly created a new patient chart electronically and identified the forms required to complete a new patient paper chart with one or less errors.	Student correctly created a new patient chart electronically and identified the forms required to complete a new patient paper chart with two errors.	Student correctly created a new patient chart electronically and identified the forms required to complete a new patient paper chart with three to four errors.	Student failed to correctly create a new patient chart electronically and was unable to successfully identify the forms required to complete a new patient paper chart or did so with five or more errors.	
Supplies and Equipment	Student obtained and had available appropriate supplies and equipment with one or less errors.	Student obtained and had available appropriate supplies and equipment with two errors.	Student obtained and had available appropriate supplies and equipment with three to four errors.	Student failed to obtain or have available appropriate supplies and equipment or did so with five or more errors.	
Medical Asepsis and Standard Precautions	Student correctly performed medical aseptic techniques and observed all required standard precautions with one or less errors.	Student correctly performed medical aseptic techniques and observed all required standard precautions with two errors.	Student correctly performed medical aseptic techniques and observed all required standard precautions with three to four errors.	Student failed to correctly perform medical aseptic techniques and observe all required standard precautions or did so with five or more errors.	
Introduction to Patient	Student appropriately introduced self to the patient with one or less errors.	Student appropriately introduced self to the patient with two errors.	Student appropriately introduced self to the patient with three to four errors.	Student failed to appropriately introduce self to the patient or did so with five or more errors.	
Obtained Intake Information	Student appropriately obtained patient intake information with one or less errors.	Student appropriately obtained patient intake information with two errors.	Student appropriately obtained patient intake information with three to four errors.	Student failed to appropriately obtain patient intake information or did so with five or more errors.	
Explanation of Procedure(s)	Student appropriately explained the procedure(s) to the patient including risks and side effects with one or less errors.	Student appropriately explained the procedure(s) including risks and side effects to the patient with two errors.	Student appropriately explained the procedure(s) including risks and side effects to the patient with three to four errors.	Student failed to appropriately explain the procedure(s) including risks and side effects to the patient or did so with five or more errors.	
Obtained Consent	Student appropriately obtained patient consent with one or less errors.	Student appropriately obtained patient consent with two errors.	Student appropriately obtained patient consent with three to four errors.	Student failed to appropriately obtain patient consent or did so with five or more errors.	

	Student performed a full patient assessment with one to two errors.	Student performed a full patient assessment with two to three errors or omitted one skill assessment.	Student performed a full patient assessment with four to five errors or omitted two skill assessments.	Student performed a full patient assessment with six or more errors or omitted three or more skills.	
Patient Assessment • **Height** • **Weight** • **Temperature** • **Pulse** • **Respiration** • **Blood Pressure**	Student performed a full patient assessment with one to two errors.	Student performed a full patient assessment with two to three errors or omitted one skill assessment.	Student performed a full patient assessment with four to five errors or omitted two skill assessments.	Student performed a full patient assessment with six or more errors or omitted three or more skills.	
Patient Instructions/ Preparation	Student provided appropriate patient instruction with one or less errors.	Student provided appropriate patient instruction with two errors.	Student provided appropriate patient instruction with three to four errors.	Student failed to provide appropriate patient instruction or did so with five or more errors.	
Supplies and Equipment Identified for the Physical Examination	Student provided the physician with the appropriate supplies and equipment with one or less errors.	Student provided the physician with the appropriate supplies and equipment with two errors.	Student provided the physician with the appropriate supplies and equipment with three to four errors.	Student failed to provide the physician with the appropriate supplies and equipment or did so with five or more errors.	
Hepatitis B Vaccine	Student properly performed the injection with one or less errors.	Student properly performed the injection with two errors.	Student properly performed the injection with three errors.	Student failed to properly perform the injection or did so with four or more errors.	
Tetanus Vaccine	Student properly performed the injection with one or less errors.	Student properly performed the injection with two errors.	Student properly performed the injection with three errors.	Student failed to properly perform the injection or did so with four or more errors.	
PPD Test	Student properly performed the injection with one or less errors.	Student properly performed the injection with two errors.	Student properly performed the injection with three errors.	Student failed to properly perform the injection or did so with four or more errors.	
Documentation	Student properly documented all procedures with one or less errors.	Student properly documented all procedures with two errors or omitted documentation of one procedure.	Student properly documented all procedures with three to four errors or omitted documentation of two procedures.	Student properly documented all procedures with five or more errors or omitted documentation of three or more procedures.	
				TOTAL	

Based on the above criteria the student's grade for this assignment is: _____

(Total the points for each element scored and average for a final grade.)

Comments to the Student:

Instructor Signature: _____ Date: _____

260

CASE STUDY 46 *Gestational Diabetes, Patient Education, and Laboratory Tests*

Name _____ Date _____

Elements	4 Excellent	3 Proficient	2 Adequate	1 Needs Improvement	Points
Medical Asepsis and Standard Precautions	Student correctly performed medical aseptic techniques and observed all required standard precautions with one or less errors.	Student correctly performed medical aseptic techniques and observed all required standard precautions with two errors.	Student correctly performed medical aseptic techniques and observed all required standard precautions with three to four errors.	Student failed to correctly perform medical aseptic techniques and observe all required standard precautions or did so with five or more errors.	
Supplies and Equipment	Student obtained and had available appropriate supplies and equipment with one or less errors.	Student obtained and had available appropriate supplies and equipment with two errors.	Student obtained and had available appropriate supplies and equipment with three to four errors.	Student failed to obtain or have available appropriate supplies and equipment or did so with five or more errors.	
Response to Question 2	Student responded appropriately to question 2 with one or less errors.	Student responded appropriately to question 2 with two errors.	Student responded appropriately to question 2 with three to four errors.	Student failed to respond appropriately to question 2 or did so with five or more errors.	
Introduction to Patient	Student appropriately introduced self to the patient with one or less errors.	Student appropriately introduced self to the patient with two errors.	Student appropriately introduced self to the patient with three to four errors.	Student failed to appropriately introduce self to the patient or did so with five or more errors.	
Obtained Intake Information	Student appropriately obtained patient intake information with one or less errors.	Student appropriately obtained patient intake information with two errors.	Student appropriately obtained patient intake information with three to four errors.	Student failed to appropriately obtain patient intake information or did so with five or more errors.	
Obtained Consent	Student appropriately obtained patient consent with one or less errors.	Student appropriately obtained patient consent with two errors.	Student appropriately obtained patient consent with three to four errors.	Student failed to appropriately obtain patient consent or did so with five or more errors.	
Patient Assessment	Student performed a full patient assessment with one to two errors.	Student performed a full patient assessment with two to three errors or omitted one skill assessment.	Student performed a full patient assessment with four to five errors or omitted two skill assessments.	Student performed a full patient assessment with six or more errors or omitted three or more skills.	
Obtain and Perform Testing on Urine Sample	Student obtained and performed a dipstick urine test with one or less errors.	Student obtained and performed a dipstick urine test with two errors.	Student obtained and performed a dipstick urine test with three to four errors.	Student failed to obtain and perform a dipstick urine test or did so with five or more errors.	
Response to Question 7	Student responded appropriately to question 7 with no errors.	Student responded appropriately to question 7 with one error.	Student responded appropriately to question 7 with two errors.	Student failed to respond appropriately to question 7 or did so with three or more errors.	

	Student appropriately assisted the physician as required with one or less errors.	Student appropriately assisted the physician as required with two errors.	Student appropriately assisted the physician as required with three to four errors.	Student failed to appropriately assist the physician as required or did so with five or more errors.	
Assisting the Physician	Student appropriately assisted the physician as required with one or less errors.	Student appropriately assisted the physician as required with two errors.	Student appropriately assisted the physician as required with three to four errors.	Student failed to appropriately assist the physician as required or did so with five or more errors.	
Response in Writing to Question 8	Student responded appropriately to question 8 with one or less errors.	Student responded appropriately to question 8 with two errors.	Student responded appropriately to question 8 with three to four errors.	Student failed to respond appropriately to question 8 or did so with five or more errors.	
Preparation of Pamphlet	Student prepared a pamphlet with three or less errors.	Student prepared a pamphlet with four errors.	Student prepared a pamphlet with five errors.	Student failed to prepare a pamphlet or did so with six or more errors.	
Explanation of Gestational Diabetes, Testing, and Healthy Nutrition	Student appropriately explained the topics with one or less errors.	Student appropriately explained the topics with two errors.	Student appropriately explained the topics with three to four errors.	Student failed to appropriately explain the topics or did so with five or more errors.	
Schedule Appointment for OGTT	Student appropriately scheduled an appointment with one or less errors.	Student appropriately scheduled an appointment with two errors.	Student appropriately scheduled an appointment with three to four errors.	Student failed to appropriately schedule an appointment or did so with five or more errors.	
Documentation	Student properly documented all procedures with one or less errors.	Student documented all procedures with two errors or omitted documentation of one procedure.	Student documented all procedures with three to four errors or omitted documentation of two procedures.	Student documented all procedures with five or more errors or omitted documentation of three or more procedures.	
				TOTAL	

Based on the above criteria the student's grade for this assignment is: _____

(Total the points for each element scored and average for a final grade.)

Comments to the Student:

Instructor Signature: _____   Date: _____

School Physicals, Patient Education, and Immunizations

Name _____ Date _____

Elements	4 Excellent	3 Proficient	2 Adequate	1 Needs Improvement	Points
New Patient Charts	Student correctly assembled new patient charts and completed all forms with one or less errors.	Student correctly assembled new patient charts and completed all forms with two errors.	Student correctly assembled new patient charts and completed all forms with three to four errors.	Student failed to correctly assemble new patient charts and/or failed to complete all forms or did so with five or more errors.	
Medical Asepsis and Standard Precautions	Student accurately performed medical aseptic techniques and observed all required standard precautions with one or less errors.	Student accurately performed medical aseptic techniques and observed all required standard precautions with two errors.	Student accurately performed medical aseptic techniques and observed all required standard precautions with three to four errors.	Student failed to accurately perform medical aseptic techniques and observe all required standard precautions or did so with five or more errors.	
Supplies and Equipment	Student provided the physician with the appropriate supplies and equipment with one or less errors.	Student provided the physician with the appropriate supplies and equipment with two errors.	Student provided the physician with the appropriate supplies and equipment with three errors.	Student failed to provide physician with the appropriate supplies and equipment or did so with four or more errors.	
Introduction to Patients	Student appropriately introduced self to the patients with one or less errors.	Student appropriately introduced self to the patients with two errors.	Student appropriately introduced self to the patients with three to four errors.	Student failed to appropriately introduce self to the patients or did so with five or more errors.	
Obtained Intake Information	Student appropriately obtained patient intake information for both patients with one or less errors.	Student appropriately obtained patient intake information for both patients with two errors.	Student appropriately obtained patient intake information for both patients with three to four errors.	Student failed to appropriately obtain patient intake information for both patients or only obtained intake information for one patient or obtained intake information for both patients with five or more errors.	
Obtained Consent	Student appropriately obtained consent with one or less errors.	Student appropriately obtained consent with two errors.	Student appropriately obtained consent with three errors.	Student failed to appropriately obtain consent or did so with four or more errors.	
Explanation of Procedure(s)	Student appropriately explained the procedure(s) to the patients with one or less errors.	Student appropriately explained the procedure(s) to the patients with two errors.	Student appropriately explained the procedure(s) to the patients with three to four errors.	Student failed to appropriately explain the procedure(s) to the patients or did so with five or more errors.	
Patient Assessment • Height • Weight • Temperature • Pulse • Respiration • Blood Pressure	Student performed a full patient assessment on both patients with one or less errors.	Student performed a full patient assessment on both patients with two errors or omitted one skill assessment.	Student performed a full patient assessment on both patients with three errors or omitted two skill assessments.	Student failed to perform a full patient assessment on both patients or performed a patient assessment with four or more errors or omitted three or more skills.	

Hearing Test	Student performed a hearing test on both patients without any errors.	Student performed a hearing test on both patients with one error.	Student performed a hearing test on both patients with two errors.	Student failed to perform a hearing test on either patient or only performed a hearing test on one patient or performed a hearing test on both patients with three or more errors.
Vision Test	Student performed a vision test on both patients without any errors.	Student performed a vision test on both patients with one error.	Student performed a vision test on both patients with two errors.	Student failed to perform a vision test on either patient or only performed a vision test on one patient or performed a vision test on both patients with three or more errors.
Patient Instructions	Student provided appropriate patient instruction with one or less errors.	Student provided appropriate patient instruction with two errors.	Student provided appropriate patient instruction with three errors.	Student failed to provide appropriate patient instruction or did so with four or more errors.
Positioning and Draping	Student properly positioned and draped the patients for a routine physical examination with no errors.	Student properly positioned and draped the patients for a routine physical examination with one error.	Student properly positioned and draped the patients for a routine physical examination with two errors.	Student failed to properly position and drape the patients or positioned and draped only one patient or positioned and draped both patients with five or more errors or positioned and draped the patients for the incorrect procedure.
Assisting the Physician	Student appropriately assisted the physician with the physical examinations with no errors.	Student assisted the physician with the physical examinations with one error.	Student assisted the physician with the physical examinations with two errors.	Student failed to assist the physician with the physical examination or assisted with only one physical examination or assisted with both physical examinations with three or more errors.
Documentation	Student properly documented all procedures with one or less errors.	Student properly documented all procedures with two errors.	Student properly documented all procedures with three errors.	Student failed to properly document all procedures or did so with four or more errors.
Response to Question 14	Student responded to the question with one or less errors.	N/A	N/A	Student failed to respond to the question or did so with two or more errors.
Response to Question 15	Student responded to the question with one or less errors.	N/A	N/A	Student failed to respond to the question or did so with two or more errors.
Explanation of Immunizations	Student appropriately explained the purposes, benefits, and risks of the immunizations to be administered with one or less errors.	Student appropriately explained the purposes, benefits, and risks of the immunizations to be administered with two errors.	Student appropriately explained the purposes, benefits, and risks of the immunizations to be administered with three to four errors.	Student failed to appropriately explain the purposes, benefits, and risks of the immunizations to be administered or did so with five or more errors.

Criteria				
Explanation of When to Return for Injection Boosters	Student explained to the parents when Tony and Nate should return for injection boosters with no errors.	N/A	N/A	Student failed to explain to the parents when Tony and Nate should return for injection boosters or did so with errors.
Immunization Preparation and Administration	Student correctly prepared and administered the appropriate immunizations with one or less errors.	Student correctly prepared and administered the appropriate immunizations with two errors.	Student correctly prepared and administered the appropriate immunizations with three errors or prepared and administered one incorrect immunization.	Student failed to correctly prepare and administer the appropriate immunizations or prepared and administered two incorrect immunizations or prepared and administered the appropriate immunizations with four or more errors.
Response to Question 18	Student appropriately responded to the question with no errors.	N/A	N/A	Student failed to respond to the question or did so with errors.
Immunization Cards	Student appropriately completed both immunization cards with one or less errors.	Student appropriately completed both immunization cards with two errors.	Student appropriately completed both immunization cards with three errors.	Student failed to appropriately complete the immunization cards or completed only one immunization card or completed both immunization cards with four or more errors.
Documentation	Student properly documented immunization procedures in the patient charts with one or less errors.	Student properly documented immunization procedures in the patient charts with two errors.	Student properly documented immunization procedures in the patient charts with three errors.	Student failed to properly document the immunization procedures in both patient charts or documented the immunization procedures in one patient chart or documented immunization procedures in the patient charts with four or more errors.
				TOTAL

Based on the above criteria the student's grade for this assignment is: _____

(Total the points for each element scored and average for a final grade.)

Comments to the Student:

Instructor Signature: _____   Date: _____

CASE STUDY 48   *First Aid—Burns*

Elements	4 Excellent	3 Proficient	2 Adequate	1 Needs Improvement	Points
New Patient Chart	Student correctly assembled a new patient chart and completed all forms with one or less errors.	Student correctly assembled a new patient chart and completed all forms with two errors.	Student correctly assembled a new patient chart and completed all forms with three errors.	Student failed to correctly assemble a new patient chart and/or failed to complete all forms or did so with four or more errors.	
Medical Asepsis and Standard Precautions	Student accurately performed medical aseptic techniques and observed all required standard precautions with one or less errors.	Student accurately performed medical aseptic techniques and observed all required standard precautions with two errors.	Student accurately performed medical aseptic techniques and observed all required standard precautions with three errors.	Student failed to accurately perform medical aseptic techniques and observe all required standard precautions or did so with four or more errors.	
Supplies and Equipment	Student assembled the appropriate supplies and equipment with one or less errors.	Student assembled the appropriate supplies and equipment with two errors.	Student assembled the appropriate supplies and equipment with three errors.	Student failed to provide the appropriate supplies and equipment or did so with four or more errors.	
Introduction to Patient	Student appropriately introduced self to the patient with no errors.	N/A	N/A	Student failed to appropriately introduce self to the patient or did so with errors.	
Obtained Intake Information	Student appropriately obtained patient intake information with no errors.	Student appropriately obtained patient intake information with one error.	Student appropriately obtained patient intake information with two errors.	Student failed to appropriately obtain patient intake information or did so with three or more errors.	
Explanation of Procedure(s)	Student appropriately explained the procedure(s) to the patient with no errors.	Student appropriately explained the procedure(s) to the patient with one error.	Student appropriately explained the procedure(s) to the patient with two errors.	Student failed to appropriately explain the procedure(s) to the patient or did so with three or more errors.	
Patient Assessment • Height • Weight • Temperature • Pulse • Respiration • Blood Pressure	Student performed a full patient assessment with one or less errors.	Student performed a full patient assessment with two errors or omitted one skill assessment.	Student performed a full patient assessment with three errors or omitted two skill assessments.	Student failed to perform a full patient assessment or did so with four or more errors or omitted three or more skills.	
Assisting the Physician	Student appropriately assisted the physician with the examination of the burns with no errors.	Student appropriately assisted the physician with the examination of the burns with one error.	Student appropriately assisted the physician with the examination of the burns with two errors.	Student failed to appropriately assist the physician with the examination of the burns or did so with three or more errors.	

Criteria					Points
Bandaging and Burn Cream Application	Student appropriately applied burn cream and bandaged the burns with no errors.	Student appropriately applied burn cream and bandaged the burns with one error.	Student appropriately applied burn cream and bandaged the burns with two errors.	Student failed to appropriately apply burn cream and bandage the burns or applied burn cream and failed to bandage the burns or applied burn cream and bandaged the burns with three or more errors.	
Patient Instruction	Student provided the patient with verbal and written instructions on caring for the burns with no errors.	Student provided the patient with verbal and written instructions on caring for the burns with one error.	Student provided the patient with verbal and written instructions on caring for the burns with two errors.	Student failed to provide the patient with verbal and written instructions on caring for the burns or did so with three or more errors.	
Pamphlet Preparation	Student prepared a patient pamphlet with one or less errors.	Student prepared a patient pamphlet with two errors.	Student prepared a patient pamphlet with three errors.	Student failed to prepare a patient pamphlet or did so with four or more errors.	
Prescription Preparation	Student accurately prepared the prescription with no errors.	Student accurately prepared the prescription with one error.	Student accurately prepared the prescription with two errors.	Student failed to accurately prepare the prescription or did so with three or more errors.	
Note Preparation	Student prepared a note stating the patient's estimated return to employment with no errors.	Student prepared a note stating the patient's estimated return to employment with one error.	Student prepared a note stating the patient's estimated return to employment with two errors.	Student failed to prepare a note stating the patient's estimated return to employment or did so with three or more errors.	
Schedule and Provide Patient with Follow-up Appointment Time	Student appropriately performed these tasks with no errors.	Student appropriately performed these tasks with one error.	Student appropriately performed these tasks with two errors.	Student failed to appropriately perform these tasks or did so with three or more errors.	
Response to Question 14	Student responded to the question with one or less errors.	N/A	N/A	Student failed to respond to the question or did so with two or more errors.	
Documentation	Student properly documented all procedures with one or less errors.	Student properly documented all procedures with two errors.	Student properly documented all procedures with three errors.	Student failed to properly document all procedures or did so with four or more errors.	
				TOTAL	

Based on the above criteria the student's grade for this assignment is: _____

(Total the points for each element scored and average for a final grade.)

Comments to the Student:

Instructor Signature: _____   Date: _____

CASE STUDY 49　　*Medication Storage*

Name _____　Date _____

Elements	4 Excellent	3 Proficient	2 Adequate	1 Needs Improvement	Points
Role-Play Scenario 1	Student participated in the role-play.	N/A	N/A	Student failed to participate in the role-play.	
Drug Classification Organization	Student accurately organized the "sample" cupboard according to drug classifications with no errors.	Student accurately organized the "sample" cupboard according to drug classifications with one error.	Student accurately organized the "sample" cupboard according to drug classifications with two errors.	Student failed to accurately organize the "sample" cupboard according to drug classifications or did so with three or more errors.	
Prescription Safekeeping Protocols	Student adhered to prescription safekeeping protocols during the organization of the cupboard.	N/A	N/A	Student failed to adhere to prescription safekeeping protocols during the organization of the cupboard.	
Top 50 Drug Classifications	Student correctly identified the top 50 drug classification categories with one or less errors.	N/A	N/A	Student failed to identify the top 50 drug classification categories or did so with two or more errors.	
Drug Category Identification	Student accurately identified three to five examples of drugs for each of the 50 drug classification categories with one or less errors.	Student accurately identified three to five examples of drugs for each of the 50 drug classification categories with two errors.	Student accurately identified three to five examples of drugs for each of the 50 drug classification categories with three errors.	Student failed to accurately identify three to five examples of drugs for each of the 50 drug classification categories or did so with four or more errors.	
Alphabetization	Student accurately alphabetized the drug classification category cards with no errors.	N/A	N/A	Student failed to accurately alphabetize the drug classification category cards or did so with errors.	
Response to Question 3	Student accurately responded to question 3 with no errors.	N/A	N/A	Student failed to accurately respond to question 3 or did so with errors.	
				TOTAL	

Based on the above criteria the student's grade for this assignment is: _____
(Total the points for each element scored and average for a final grade.)

Comments to the Student:

Instructor Signature: _____　Date: _____

CASE STUDY 50 *Allergy Testing*

Name _____ Date _____

Elements	4 Excellent	3 Proficient	2 Adequate	1 Needs Improvement	Points
Medical Asepsis and Standard Precautions	Student correctly performed medical aseptic techniques and observed all required standard precautions with one or less errors.	Student correctly performed medical aseptic techniques and observed all required standard precautions with two errors.	Student correctly performed medical aseptic techniques and observed all required standard precautions with three to four errors.	Student failed to correctly perform medical aseptic techniques and observe standard precautions or did so with five or more errors.	
Supplies and Equipment	Student obtained and had available appropriate supplies and equipment with one or less errors.	Student obtained and had available appropriate supplies and equipment with two errors.	Student obtained and had available appropriate supplies and equipment with three to four errors.	Student failed to obtain or have available appropriate supplies and equipment or did so with five or more errors.	
Introduction to Patient	Student appropriately introduced self to the patient with one or less errors.	Student appropriately introduced self to the patient with two errors.	Student appropriately introduced self to the patient with three to four errors.	Student failed to appropriately introduce self to the patient or did so with five or more errors.	
Obtained Intake Information	Student appropriately obtained patient intake information with one or less errors.	Student appropriately obtained patient intake information with two errors.	Student appropriately obtained patient intake information with three to four errors.	Student failed to appropriately obtain patient intake information or did so with five or more errors.	
Explanation of Procedure(s)	Student provided appropriate explanation, including the risks and normal and abnormal reactions, with one or less errors.	Student provided appropriate explanation, including the risks and normal and abnormal reactions, with two errors.	Student provided appropriate explanation, including the risks and normal and abnormal reactions, with three to four errors.	Student failed to provide appropriate explanation, including the risks and normal and abnormal reactions, or did so with five or more errors.	
Obtained Consent	Student appropriately obtained patient consent with one or less errors.	Student appropriately obtained patient consent with two errors.	Student appropriately obtained patient consent with three to four errors.	Student failed to appropriately obtain patient consent or did so with five or more errors.	
Patient Assessment • **Height** • **Weight** • **Temperature** • **Pulse** • **Respiration** • **Blood Pressure**	Student performed a full patient assessment with one to two errors.	Student performed a full patient assessment with two to three errors or omitted one skill assessment.	Student performed a full patient assessment with four to five errors or omitted two skill assessments.	Student performed a full patient assessment with six or more errors or omitted three or more skills.	
Patient Instructions	Student provided appropriate patient instruction with one or less errors.	Student provided appropriate patient instruction with two errors.	Student provided appropriate patient instruction with three to four errors.	Student failed to provide appropriate patient instruction or did so with five or more errors.	
Allergy Skin Test 1	Student properly performed the intradermal injection with one or less errors.	Student properly performed the intradermal injection with two errors.	Student properly performed the intradermal injection with three errors.	Student failed to properly perform the intradermal injection or did so with four or more errors.	

Criteria					
Allergy Skin Test 2	Student properly performed the intradermal injection with one or less errors.	Student properly performed the intradermal injection with two errors.	Student properly performed the intradermal injection with three errors.	Student failed to properly perform the intradermal injection or did so with four or more errors.	
Allergy Skin Test 3	Student properly performed the intradermal injection with one or less errors.	Student properly performed the intradermal injection with two errors.	Student properly performed the intradermal injection with three errors.	Student failed to properly perform the intradermal injection or did so with four or more errors.	
Allergy Skin Test 4	Student properly performed the intradermal injection with one or less errors.	Student properly performed the intradermal injection with two errors.	Student properly performed the intradermal injection with three errors.	Student failed to properly perform the intradermal injection or did so with four or more errors.	
Allergy Injection First Dose	Student properly performed the subcutaneous injection with one or less errors.	Student properly performed the subcutaneous injection with two errors.	Student properly performed the subcutaneous injection with three errors.	Student failed to properly perform the subcutaneous injection or did so with four or more errors.	
Allergy Injection Second Dose	Student properly performed the subcutaneous injection with one or less errors.	Student properly performed the subcutaneous injection with two errors.	Student properly performed the subcutaneous injection with three errors.	Student failed to properly perform the subcutaneous injection or did so with four or more errors.	
Allergy Injection Third Dose	Student properly performed the subcutaneous injection with one or less errors.	Student properly performed the subcutaneous injection with two errors.	Student properly performed the subcutaneous injection with three errors.	Student failed to properly perform the subcutaneous injection or did so with four or more errors.	
Response to Question 11	Student responded appropriately to question 11 with one or less errors.	Student responded appropriately to question 11 with two errors.	Student responded appropriately to question 11 with three to four errors.	Student failed to respond appropriately to question 11 or did so with five or more errors.	
Response to Question 12	Student responded appropriately to question 12 with one or less errors.	Student responded appropriately to question 12 with two errors.	Student responded appropriately to question 12 with three to four errors.	Student failed to respond appropriately to question 12 or did so with five or more errors.	
Documentation	Student properly documented all procedures with one or less errors.	Student properly documented all procedures with two errors or omitted documentation of one procedure.	Student properly documented all procedures with three to four errors or omitted documentation of two procedures.	Student properly documented all procedures with five or more errors or omitted documentation of three or more procedures.	
				TOTAL	

Based on the above criteria the student's grade for this assignment is: _____

(Total the points for each element scored and average for a final grade.)

Comments to the Student:

Instructor Signature: _____   Date: _____

First Aid–Bleeding

Name _____ Date _____

Elements	4 Excellent	3 Proficient	2 Adequate	1 Needs Improvement	Points
Medical Asepsis and Standard Precautions	Student accurately performed medical aseptic techniques and observed all required standard precautions with one or less errors.	Student accurately performed medical aseptic techniques and observed all required standard precautions with two errors.	Student accurately performed medical aseptic techniques and observed all required standard precautions with three errors.	Student failed to accurately perform medical aseptic techniques and observe all required standard precautions or did so with four or more errors.	
Supplies and Equipment	Student assembled the appropriate supplies and equipment with one or less errors.	Student assembled the appropriate supplies and equipment with two errors.	Student assembled the appropriate supplies and equipment with three errors.	Student failed to provide the appropriate supplies and equipment or did so with four or more errors.	
Introduction to Patient	Student appropriately introduced self to the patient with no errors.	N/A	N/A	Student failed to appropriately introduce self to the patient or did so with errors.	
Establishing a Rapport	Student properly established a rapport with the patient with no errors.	Student properly established a rapport with the patient with one error.	Student properly established a rapport with the patient with two errors.	Student failed to properly establish a rapport with the patient or did so with three or more errors.	
Obtained Intake Information	Student appropriately obtained patient intake information with no errors.	Student appropriately obtained patient intake information with one error.	Student appropriately obtained patient intake information with two errors.	Student failed to appropriately obtain patient intake information or did so with three or more errors.	
Patient Assessment • Height • Weight • Temperature • Pulse • Respiration • Blood Pressure	Student performed a full patient assessment with one or less errors.	Student performed a full patient assessment with two errors or omitted one skill assessment.	Student performed a full patient assessment with three errors or omitted two skill assessments.	Student failed to perform a full patient assessment or did so with four or more errors or omitted three or more skills.	
Pressure Point	Student lifted the patient's leg and used the correct pressure point with no errors.	Student lifted the patient's leg and used the correct pressure point with one error.	Student lifted the patient's leg and used the correct pressure point with two errors.	Student failed to lift the leg and use the correct pressure point or did so with three or more errors.	
Requesting Assistance	Student requested assistance with the patient's leg and pressure point.	N/A	N/A	Student failed to ask for assistance with the patient's leg and pressure point.	

Criteria				
Supplies and Equipment	Student accurately identified the supplies and equipment necessary for the surgical repair of a laceration with one or less errors.	Student accurately identified the supplies and equipment necessary for the surgical repair of a laceration with two errors.	Student accurately identified the supplies and equipment necessary for the surgical repair of a laceration with three errors.	Student failed to accurately identify the supplies and equipment necessary for the surgical repair of a laceration or did so with four or more errors.
Preparing Room for Surgical Procedure	Student accurately prepared the room for a surgical repair of a laceration with one or less errors.	Student accurately prepared the room for a surgical repair of a laceration with two errors.	Student accurately prepared the room for a surgical repair of a laceration with three errors.	Student failed to accurately prepare the room for a surgical repair of a laceration or did so with four or more errors.
Role-Play the Conversation with Physician	Student accurately informed Dr. Bledsole of the patient's current condition with no errors.	N/A	N/A	Student failed to accurately inform Dr. Bledsole of the patient's current condition or did so with errors.
Injection	Student accurately calculated, prepared, and administered the appropriate dose of ketamine and atropine with no errors.	Student accurately calculated, prepared, and administered the appropriate dose of ketamine and atropine with one error.	Student accurately calculated, prepared, and administered the appropriate dose of ketamine and atropine with two errors.	Student failed to accurately calculate, prepare, and administer the appropriate dose of ketamine and atropine or did so with three or more errors.
Preparing Equipment for Surgery	Student opened the necessary sterile packs and equipment required for the repair with no errors.	N/A	N/A	Student failed to open the necessary sterile packs and equipment required for the repair or did so with errors.
Surgical Scrub and Draping	Student performed a surgical scrub and wound draping with no errors.	Student performed a surgical scrub and wound draping with one error.	Student performed a surgical scrub and wound draping with two errors.	Student failed to perform a surgical scrub or wound draping or performed a surgical scrub and wound draping with three or more errors.
Assisting the Physician	Student appropriately assisted the physician with the laceration repair with no errors.	Student appropriately assisted the physician with the laceration repair with one error.	Student appropriately assisted the physician with the laceration repair with two errors.	Student failed to appropriately assist the physician with the laceration repair or did so with three or more errors.
Pulse and Respiration Monitoring	Student monitored the patient's pulse and respiration during the procedure with no errors.	N/A	N/A	Student failed to monitor the patient's pulse and respiration during the procedure or did so with errors.
Dressing Application	Student accurately applied dressings to the sutured wound with no errors.	N/A	N/A	Student failed to apply dressings to the sutured wound or did so with errors.
Patient Instruction	Student provided the patient's mother with verbal and written instructions regarding the care of sutures and lacerations with one or less errors.	Student provided the patient's mother with verbal and written instructions regarding the care of sutures and lacerations with two errors.	Student provided the patient's mother with verbal and written instructions regarding the care of sutures and lacerations with three errors.	Student failed to provide the patient's mother with verbal and written instructions regarding the care of sutures and lacerations or did so with four or more errors.

Telephoning Prescription Orders	Student accurately telephoned in a pain medication for the patient with no errors.	Student accurately telephoned in a pain medication for the patient with one error.	Student accurately telephoned in a pain medication for the patient with two errors.	Student failed to accurately telephone in a pain medication for the patient or did so with three or more errors.	
Documentation	Student properly documented all procedures and entered the information into the patient's electronic medical record with one or less errors.	Student properly documented all procedures and entered the information into the patient's electronic medical record with two errors.	Student properly documented all procedures and entered the information into the patient's electronic medical record with three errors.	Student failed to properly document all procedures or failed to enter the information into the patient's electronic medical record or documented all procedures and entered the information into the patient's electronic medical record with four or more errors.	
Surgical Pack Preparation	Student accurately prepared the surgical packs for sterilization with one or less errors.	Student accurately prepared the surgical packs for sterilization with two errors.	Student accurately prepared the surgical packs for sterilization with three errors.	Student failed to accurately prepare the surgical packs for sterilization or did so with four or more errors.	
Restocking Equipment and Supplies	Student restocked the necessary equipment and supplies with no errors.	N/A	N/A	Student failed to restock the necessary equipment and supplies or did so with errors.	
				TOTAL	

Based on the above criteria the student's grade for this assignment is: _____

(Total the points for each element scored and average for a final grade.)

Comments to the Student:

Instructor Signature: _____   Date: _____

CASE STUDY 52 *Hypertensive Emergency*

Name _____ Date _____

Elements	4 Excellent	3 Proficient	2 Adequate	1 Needs Improvement	Points
Introduction to Patient	Student appropriately introduced self to the patient with one or less errors.	Student appropriately introduced self to the patient with two errors.	Student appropriately introduced self to the patient with three to four errors.	Student failed to appropriately introduce self to the patient or did so with five or more errors.	
Medical Asepsis and Standard Precautions	Student correctly performed medical aseptic techniques and observed all required standard precautions with one or less errors.	Student correctly performed medical aseptic techniques and observed all required standard precautions with two errors.	Student correctly performed medical aseptic techniques and observed all required standard precautions with three to four errors.	Student failed to correctly perform medical aseptic techniques and observe all required standard precautions or did so with five or more errors.	
Supplies and Equipment	Student obtained and had available appropriate supplies and equipment with one or less errors.	Student obtained and had available appropriate supplies and equipment with two errors.	Student obtained and had available appropriate supplies and equipment with three to four errors.	Student failed to obtain or have available appropriate supplies and equipment or did so with five or more errors.	
Obtain Patient Intake Information	Student appropriately obtained patient intake information with one or less errors.	Student appropriately obtained patient intake information with two errors.	Student appropriately obtained patient intake information with three to four errors.	Student failed to appropriately obtain patient intake information or did so with five or more errors.	
Obtained Consent	Student appropriately obtained patient consent with one or less errors.	Student appropriately obtained patient consent with two errors.	Student appropriately obtained patient consent with three to four errors.	Student failed to appropriately obtain patient consent or did so with five or more errors.	
Patient Assessment • Height • Weight • Temperature • Pulse • Respiration • Blood Pressure	Student performed a full patient assessment with one to two errors.	Student performed a full patient assessment with two to three errors or omitted one skill assessment.	Student performed a full patient assessment with four to five errors or omitted two skill assessments.	Student performed a full patient assessment with six or more errors or omitted three or more skills.	
Administering Oxygen by Cannula	Student correctly demonstrated this task with no errors.	Student correctly demonstrated this task with one error.	Student correctly demonstrated this task with two errors.	Student failed to correctly demonstrate this task or did so with three or more errors.	
Explanation of Disrobing, Gowning, and Draping	Student appropriately explained how to disrobe, gown, and drape for the procedures with one or less errors.	Student appropriately explained how to disrobe, gown, and drape for the procedures with two errors.	Student appropriately explained how to disrobe, gown, and drape for the procedures with three to four errors.	Student failed to appropriately explain how to disrobe, gown, and drape for the procedures or did so with five or more errors.	
Assisting the Physician	Student appropriately assisted the physician as required with one or less errors.	Student appropriately assisted the physician as required with two errors.	Student appropriately assisted the physician as required with three to four errors.	Student failed to appropriately assist the physician as required or did so with five or more errors.	

	Student properly performed an ECG with one or less errors.	Student properly performed an ECG with two errors.	Student properly performed an ECG with three to four errors.	Student failed to properly perform an ECG or did so with five or more errors.	
Perform Electrocardiography	Student properly performed an ECG with one or less errors.	Student properly performed an ECG with two errors.	Student properly performed an ECG with three to four errors.	Student failed to properly perform an ECG or did so with five or more errors.	
Notifying Emergency Services	Student notified Emergency Services and provided them with the correct information while maintaining professional communication and behavior.	N/A	N/A	Student failed to notify Emergency Services or notified Emergency Services while maintaining professional communication techniques and omitted relevant information or notified Emergency Services and provided them with the correct information without demonstrating appropriate professional communication and behavior.	
Patient Explanation and Preparation for Transport	Student appropriately explained the situation and prepared the patient for transport with one or less errors.	Student appropriately explained the situation and prepared the patient for transport with two errors.	Student appropriately explained the situation and prepared the patient for transport with three to four errors.	Student failed to appropriately explain the situation or prepare the patient for transport or did so with five or more errors.	
Documentation	Student properly documented all procedures with one or less errors.	Student properly documented all with two errors or omitted documentation of one procedure.	Student properly documented all with two errors or omitted documentation of one procedure.	Student properly documented all procedures with five or more errors or omitted documentation of three or more procedures.	
Research Report	Student researched and developed a quality report with one or less errors.	Student researched and developed a quality report with two errors.	Student researched and developed a quality report with three to four errors.	Student failed to research and develop a quality report or did so with five or more errors.	
Responding to Emergency Walk-In Patient	Student appropriately responded to an emergency walk-in patient with no errors.	Student appropriately responded to an emergency walk-in patient with one error.	Student appropriately responded to an emergency walk-in patient with two to three errors.	Student failed to appropriately respond to an emergency walk-in patient or did so with four or more errors.	
				TOTAL	

Based on the above criteria the student's grade for this assignment is: _____
(Total the points for each element scored and average for a final grade.)

Comments to the Student:

Instructor Signature: _____   Date: _____

Choking, Pediatric

Name _____ Date _____

Elements	4 Excellent	3 Proficient	2 Adequate	1 Needs Improvement	Points
Role-Play Scenario 1	Student participated in the role-play scenario.	N/A	N/A	Student failed to participate in the role-play scenario.	
Patient Greeting	Student appropriately greeted the patient at the front desk.	N/A	N/A	Student failed to appropriately greet the patient at the front desk.	
Responding to an Emergency	Student appropriately responded to an emergency with no errors.	Student appropriately responded to an emergency with one error.	Student appropriately responded to an emergency with two to three errors.	Student failed to appropriately respond to an emergency or did so with four or more errors.	
Assessment and Triage	Student accurately assessed and triaged the patient with one or less errors.	Student accurately assessed and triaged the patient with two errors.	Student accurately assessed and triaged the patient with three to four errors.	Student failed to assess and triage the patient or did so with five or more errors.	
Heimlich Maneuver	Student accurately performed abdominal thrusts with no errors.	Student accurately performed abdominal thrusts with one error.	Student accurately performed abdominal thrusts with two errors.	Student failed to accurately perform abdominal thrusts or did so with three or more errors.	
Patient Assessment • Pulse • Respiration	Student performed a patient assessment to include pulse and respiration after performing abdominal thrusts with no errors.	Student performed a patient assessment to include pulse and respiration after performing abdominal thrusts with one error.	Student performed a patient assessment to include pulse and respiration after performing abdominal thrusts with two errors.	Student failed to perform a patient assessment to include pulse and respiration after performing abdominal thrusts or did so with three or more errors.	
Response to Question 3	Student responded appropriately to question 3 with one or less errors.	Student responded appropriately to question 3 with two errors.	Student responded appropriately to question 3 with three errors.	Student failed to respond appropriately to question 3 or did so with four or more errors.	
Documentation	Student properly documented the occurrence on a SOAP Note form with no errors.	Student properly documented the occurrence on a SOAP Note form with one error.	Student properly documented the occurrence on a SOAP Note form with two errors.	Student failed to properly document the occurrence on a SOAP Note form or did so with three or more errors.	
				TOTAL	

Based on the above criteria the student's grade for this assignment is: _____
(Total the points for each element scored and average for a final grade.)

Comments to the Student:

Instructor Signature: _____ Date: _____

Respiratory Distress

Name _____ Date _____

Elements	4 Excellent	3 Proficient	2 Adequate	1 Needs Improvement	Points
Medical Asepsis and Standard Precautions	Student accurately performed medical aseptic techniques and observed all required standard precautions with one or less errors.	Student accurately performed medical aseptic techniques and observed all required standard precautions with two errors.	Student accurately performed medical aseptic techniques and observed all required standard precautions with three to four errors.	Student failed to accurately perform medical aseptic techniques and observe all required standard precautions or did so with five or more errors.	
Supplies and Equipment	Student assembled the appropriate supplies and equipment with one or less errors.	Student assembled the appropriate supplies and equipment with two errors.	Student assembled the appropriate supplies and equipment with three errors.	Student failed to provide the appropriate supplies and equipment or did so with four or more errors.	
Introduction to Patient	Student appropriately introduced self to the patient with no errors.	N/A	N/A	Student failed to appropriately introduce self to the patient or did so with errors.	
Obtained Intake Information	Student appropriately obtained patient intake information with no errors.	Student appropriately obtained patient intake information with one error.	Student appropriately obtained patient intake information with two errors.	Student failed to appropriately obtain patient intake information or did so with three or more errors.	
Explanation of Procedure(s)	Student appropriately explained the procedure(s) to the patient with one or less errors.	Student appropriately explained the procedure(s) to the patient with two errors.	Student appropriately explained the procedure(s) to the patient with three errors.	Student failed to appropriately explain the procedure(s) to the patient or did so with four or more errors.	
Patient Assessment • Height • Weight • Temperature • Pulse • Respiration • Blood Pressure	Student performed a full patient assessment with no errors.	Student performed a full patient assessment with one error.	Student performed a full patient assessment with two errors or omitted one skill assessment.	Student failed to perform a full patient assessment or performed a patient assessment with three or more errors or omitted two or more skills.	
Pulse Oximetry	Student accurately performed pulse oximetry testing with no errors.	Student accurately performed pulse oximetry testing with one error.	Student accurately performed pulse oximetry testing with two errors.	Student failed to accurately perform pulse oximetry testing or did so with three or more errors.	
Response to Question 7	Student accurately responded to question 7 with no errors.	N/A	N/A	Student failed to accurately respond to question 7 or did so with errors.	
Spirometry	Student accurately performed spirometry testing with no errors.	Student accurately performed spirometry testing with one error.	Student accurately performed spirometry testing with two errors.	Student failed to accurately perform spirometry testing or did so with three or more errors.	
Response to Question 8	Student accurately responded to question 8 with no errors.	N/A	N/A	Student failed to accurately respond to question 8 or did so with errors.	
Nebulizer Treatment	Student accurately prepared and administered a nebulizer treatment with one or less errors.	Student accurately prepared and administered a nebulizer treatment with two errors.	Student accurately prepared and administered a nebulizer treatment with three errors.	Student failed to accurately prepare and administer a nebulizer treatment or did so with four or more errors.	

Schedule Chest X-ray	Student accurately scheduled a chest X-ray for the patient with no errors.	N/A	N/A	Student failed to accurately schedule a chest X-ray for the patient or did so with errors.
Patient Escort	Student escorted the patient to the laboratory.	N/A	N/A	Student failed to escort the patient to the laboratory.
Patient Hospital Admission	Student telephoned the hospital to admit the patient with no errors.	N/A	N/A	Student failed to telephone the hospital to admit the patient or did so with errors.
Documentation Collection	Student obtained the necessary information for patient admission to the hospital with no errors.	Student obtained the necessary information for patient admission to the hospital with one error.	Student obtained the necessary information for patient admission to the hospital with two errors.	Student failed to obtain the necessary information for patient admission to the hospital or did so with three or more errors.
Documentation	Student properly documented all procedures and results on a SOAP Note form and within the patient's electronic chart with one or less errors.	Student documented all procedures and results on a SOAP Note form and within the patient's electronic chart with two errors.	Student documented all procedures and results on a SOAP Note form and within the patient's electronic chart with three errors.	Student failed to document all procedures and results on a SOAP Note form or within the patient's electronic chart or did so with four or more errors.
Coding	Student accurately coded the procedures with no errors.	Student accurately coded the procedures with one error.	Student accurately coded the procedures with two errors.	Student failed to accurately code the procedures or did so with three or more errors.
Preparing Claim Form	Student accurately completed a claim form with no errors.	Student accurately completed a claim form with one error.	Student accurately completed a claim form with two errors.	Student failed to accurately complete a claim form or did so with three or more errors.
Prepare Claim Form for Mailing	Student accurately readied the claim form for the mail with no errors.	N/A	N/A	Student failed to accurately ready the claim form for the mail or did so with errors.
				TOTAL

Based on the above criteria the student's grade for this assignment is: _____

(Total the points for each element scored and average for a final grade.)

Comments to the Student:

Instructor Signature: _____ Date: _____

Electrocardiography, Venipuncture

Name _____ Date _____

Elements	4 Excellent	3 Proficient	2 Adequate	1 Needs Improvement	Points
Medical Asepsis and Standard Precautions	Student correctly performed medical aseptic techniques and observed all required standard precautions with one or less errors.	Student correctly performed medical aseptic techniques and observed all required standard precautions with two errors.	Student correctly performed medical aseptic techniques and observed all required standard precautions with three to four errors.	Student failed to correctly perform medical aseptic techniques and observe all required standard precautions or did so with five or more errors.	
Supplies and Equipment	Student obtained and had available appropriate supplies and equipment with one or less errors.	Student obtained and had available appropriate supplies and equipment with two errors.	Student obtained and had available appropriate supplies and equipment with three to four errors.	Student failed to obtain or have available appropriate supplies and equipment or did so with five or more errors.	
Introduction to Patient	Student appropriately introduced self to the patient with one or less errors.	Student appropriately introduced self to the patient with two errors.	Student appropriately introduced self to the patient with three to four errors.	Student failed to appropriately introduce self to the patient or did so with five or more errors.	
Obtained Intake Information	Student appropriately obtained patient intake information with one or less errors.	Student appropriately obtained patient intake information with two errors.	Student appropriately obtained patient intake information with three to four errors.	Student failed to appropriately obtain patient intake information or did so with five or more errors.	
Explanation of Procedure(s)	Student appropriately explained the procedure(s) to the patient with one or less errors.	Student appropriately explained the procedure(s) to the patient with two errors.	Student appropriately explained the procedure(s) to the patient with three to four errors.	Student failed to appropriately explain the procedure(s) to the patient or did so with five or more errors.	
Obtained Consent	Student appropriately obtained patient consent with one or less errors.	Student appropriately obtained patient consent with two errors.	Student appropriately obtained patient consent with three to four errors.	Student failed to appropriately obtain patient consent or did so with five or more errors.	
Patient Assessment • Height • Weight • Temperature • Pulse • Respiration • Blood Pressure	Student performed a full patient assessment with one to two errors.	Student performed a full patient assessment with two to three errors or omitted one skill assessment.	Student performed a full patient assessment with four to five errors or omitted two skill assessments.	Student performed a full patient assessment with six or more errors or omitted three or more skills.	
Patient Instructions	Student provided appropriate patient instruction with one or less errors.	Student provided appropriate patient instruction with two errors.	Student provided appropriate patient instruction with three to four errors.	Student failed to provide appropriate patient instruction or did so with five or more errors.	
Perform Electrocardiography	Student properly performed an ECG with one or less errors.	Student properly performed an ECG with two errors.	Student properly performed an ECG with three to four errors.	Student failed to appropriately perform an ECG or did so with five or more errors.	

Perform Venipuncture	Student properly performed a venipuncture with one or less errors.	Student properly performed a venipuncture with two errors.	Student properly performed a venipuncture with three to four errors.	Student failed to properly perform a venipuncture or did so with five or more errors.	
Correct Number and Color-Topped Tubes	Student obtained blood in the correct number and color-topped tubes with one or less errors.	Student obtained blood in the correct number and color-topped tubes with two errors.	Student obtained blood in the correct number and color-topped tubes with three to four errors.	Student failed to obtain blood in the correct number and color-topped tubes or did so with five or more errors.	
Package Specimens for Laboratory	Student properly packaged the specimens to be sent to the laboratory with one or less errors.	Student properly packaged the specimens to be sent to the laboratory with two errors.	Student properly packaged the specimens to be sent to the laboratory with three to four errors.	Student failed to properly package the specimens to be sent to the laboratory or did so with five or more errors.	
Response to Question 17	Student responded appropriately to question 17 with one or less errors.	Student responded appropriately to question 17 with two errors.	Student responded appropriately to question 17 with three to four errors.	Student failed to respond appropriately to question 17 or did so with five or more errors.	
Response to Question 18	Student responded appropriately to question 18 with one or less errors.	Student responded appropriately to question 18 with two errors.	Student responded appropriately to question 18 with three to four errors.	Student failed to respond appropriately to question 18 or did so with five or more errors.	
Response to Question 19	Student responded appropriately to question 19 with one or less errors.	Student responded appropriately to question 19 with two errors.	Student responded appropriately to question 19 with three to four errors.	Student failed to respond appropriately to question 19 or did so with five or more errors.	
Documentation	Student properly documented all procedures with one or less errors.	Student properly documented procedures with two errors or omitted documentation of one procedure.	Student properly documented procedures with three to four errors or omitted documentation of two procedures.	Student failed to properly document procedures or did so with five or more errors.	
				TOTAL	

Based on the above criteria the student's grade for this assignment is: _____

(Total the points for each element scored and average for a final grade.)

Comments to the Student:

Instructor Signature: _____   Date: _____

CASE STUDY 56

Urinalysis, Catheterization, and Communication Barriers

Name _____   Date _____

Elements	4 Excellent	3 Proficient	2 Adequate	1 Needs Improvement	Points
New Patient Chart	Student correctly assembled a new patient chart and completed all forms with one or less errors.	Student correctly assembled a new patient chart and completed all forms with two errors.	Student correctly assembled a new patient chart and completed all forms with three to four errors.	Student failed to correctly assemble a new patient chart and/or failed to complete all forms or did so with five or more errors.	
Medical Asepsis and Standard Precautions	Student correctly performed medical aseptic techniques and observed all required standard precautions with one or less errors.	Student correctly performed medical aseptic techniques and observed all required standard precautions with two errors.	Student correctly performed medical aseptic techniques and observed all required standard precautions with three to four errors.	Student failed to correctly perform medical aseptic techniques and observe all required standard precautions or did so with five or more errors.	
Supplies and Equipment	Student obtained and had available appropriate supplies and equipment with one or less errors.	Student obtained and had available appropriate supplies and equipment with two errors.	Student obtained and had available appropriate supplies and equipment with three to four errors.	Student failed to obtain or have available appropriate supplies and equipment or did so with five or more errors.	
Response to Question 3	Student responded appropriately to question 3 with one or less errors.	Student responded appropriately to question 3 with two errors.	Student responded appropriately to question 3 with three to four errors.	Student failed to respond appropriately to question 3 or did so with five or more errors.	
Introduction to Patient	Student appropriately introduced self to the patient with one or less errors.	Student appropriately introduced self to the patient with two errors.	Student appropriately introduced self to the patient with three to four errors.	Student failed to appropriately introduce self to the patient or did so with five or more errors.	
Obtained Intake Information	Student appropriately obtained patient intake information with one or less errors.	Student appropriately obtained patient intake information with two errors.	Student appropriately obtained patient intake information with three to four errors.	Student failed to appropriately obtain patient intake information or did so with five or more errors.	
Obtained Consent	Student appropriately obtained patient consent with one or less errors.	Student appropriately obtained patient consent with two errors.	Student appropriately obtained patient consent with three to four errors.	Student failed to appropriately obtain patient consent or did so with five or more errors.	
Patient Assessment	Student performed a full patient assessment with one to two errors.	Student performed a full patient assessment with two to three errors or omitted one skill assessment.	Student performed a full patient assessment with four to five errors or omitted two skill assessments.	Student performed a full patient assessment with six or more errors or omitted three or more skills.	
Response to Question 7	Student responded appropriately to question 7 with one or less errors.	Student responded appropriately to question 7 with two errors.	Student responded appropriately to question 7 with three to four errors.	Student failed to respond appropriately to question 7 or did so with five or more errors.	

Criterion				
Perform Venipuncture	Student properly performed a venipuncture with one or less errors.	Student properly performed a venipuncture with two errors.	Student properly performed a venipuncture with three to four errors.	Student failed to properly perform a venipuncture or did so with five or more errors.
Correct Number and Color-Topped Tubes Identified Correct Order of Draw	Student obtained blood in the correct number and color-topped tubes and identified the correct order of draw with one or less errors.	Student obtained blood in the correct number and color-topped tubes and identified the correct order of draw with two errors.	Student obtained blood in the correct number and color-topped tubes and identified the correct order of draw with three to four errors.	Student failed to obtain blood in the correct number and color-topped tubes and identified the correct order of draw or did so with five or more errors.
Package Specimens for Laboratory (Specimens were properly collected and labeled)	Student properly packaged the specimens to be sent to the laboratory with one or less errors.	Student properly packaged the specimens to be sent to the laboratory with two errors.	Student properly packaged the specimens to be sent to the laboratory with three to four errors.	Student failed to properly package the specimens to be sent to the laboratory or did so with five or more errors.
Perform CBC with ESR	Student properly performed a CBC and ESR with one or less errors.	Student properly performed a CBC and ESR with two errors.	Student properly performed a CBC and ESR with three to four errors.	Student failed to perform a CBC and ESR or did so with five or more errors.
Explanation of Disrobing, Gowning, and Draping	Student appropriately explained how to disrobe, gown, and drape for the procedures with one or less errors.	Student appropriately explained how to disrobe, gown, and drape for the procedures with two errors.	Student appropriately explained how to disrobe, gown, and drape for the procedures with three to four errors.	Student failed to appropriately explain how to disrobe, gown, and drape for the procedures or did so with five or more errors.
Explanation of Foley Catheterization	Student appropriately explained how a Foley catheterization procedure works with one or less errors.	Student appropriately explained how a Foley catheterization procedure works with two errors.	Student appropriately explained how a Foley catheterization procedure works with three to four errors.	Student failed to appropriately explain how a Foley catheterization procedure works or did so with five or more errors.
Response in Writing to Question 10	Student responded appropriately to question 10 with one or less errors.	Student responded appropriately to question 10 with two errors.	Student responded appropriately to question 10 with three to four errors.	Student failed to respond appropriately to question 10 or did so with five or more errors.
Assisting the Physician with Foley Catheterization	Student appropriately assisted the physician as required with one or less errors.	Student appropriately assisted the physician as required with two errors.	Student appropriately assisted the physician as required with three to four errors.	Student failed to appropriately assist the physician as required or did so with five or more errors.
Response in Writing to Question 12	Student responded appropriately to question 12 with no errors.	Student responded appropriately to question 12 with one error.	Student responded appropriately to question 12 with two errors.	Student failed to respond appropriately to question 12 or did so with three or more errors.
Perform a Full Urinalysis	Student properly performed a full urinalysis with one or less errors.	Student properly performed a full urinalysis with two errors.	Student properly performed a full urinalysis with three to four errors.	Student failed to properly perform a full urinalysis or did so with five or more errors.
Explanation of Catheter Leg Bag Procedure	Student appropriately explained the procedure to the patient with one or less errors.	Student appropriately explained the procedure to the patient with two errors.	Student appropriately explained the procedure to the patient with three to four errors.	Student failed to appropriately explain the procedure to the patient or did so with five or more errors.

	Student correctly completed the prescription with one or less errors.	Student correctly completed the prescription with two errors.	Student correctly completed the prescription with three to four errors.	Student failed to correctly complete the prescription or did so with five or more errors.	
Prescription	Student correctly completed the prescription with one or less errors.	Student correctly completed the prescription with two errors.	Student correctly completed the prescription with three to four errors.	Student failed to correctly complete the prescription or did so with five or more errors.	
Assisting the Physician with Catheter Leg Bag	Student appropriately assisted the physician as required with one or less errors.	Student appropriately assisted the physician as required with two errors.	Student appropriately assisted the physician as required with three to four errors.	Student failed to appropriately assist the physician as required or did so with five or more errors.	
Explanation about Possible Symptoms and Follow-up Appointment	Student appropriately explained the possible symptoms and follow-up appointment to the patient with one or less errors.	Student appropriately explained the possible symptoms and follow-up appointment to the patient with two errors.	Student appropriately explained the possible symptoms and follow-up appointment to the patient with three to four errors.	Student failed to appropriately explain the possible symptoms and follow-up appointment to the patient or did so with five or more errors.	
Communication	Student appropriately communicated with a non-English-speaking patient.	N/A	N/A	Student failed to appropriately communicate with a non-English-speaking patient.	
Documentation	Student properly documented all procedures with one or less errors.	Student properly documented all procedures with two errors or omitted documentation of one procedure.	Student properly documented all procedures with three to four errors or omitted documentation of two procedures.	Student properly documented all procedures with five or more errors or omitted documentation of three or more procedures.	
					TOTAL

Based on the above criteria the student's grade for this assignment is: _____

(Total the points for each element scored and average for a final grade.)

Comments to the Student:

Instructor Signature: _____   Date: _____

Fracture

Name _____ Date _____

Elements	4 Excellent	3 Proficient	2 Adequate	1 Needs Improvement	Points
Response to Question 2	Student responded appropriately to question 2 with one or less errors.	Student responded appropriately to question 2 with two errors.	Student responded appropriately to question 2 with three to four errors.	Student failed to respond appropriately to question 2 or did so with five or more errors.	
Medical Asepsis and Standard Precautions	Student correctly performed medical aseptic techniques and observed all required standard precautions with one or less errors.	Student correctly performed medical aseptic techniques and observed all required standard precautions with two errors.	Student correctly performed medical aseptic techniques and observed all required standard precautions with three to four errors.	Student failed to correctly perform medical aseptic techniques and observe all required standard precautions or did so with five or more errors.	
Supplies and Equipment	Student obtained and had available appropriate supplies and equipment with one or less errors.	Student obtained and had available appropriate supplies and equipment with two errors.	Student obtained and had available appropriate supplies and equipment with three to four errors.	Student failed to obtain or have available appropriate supplies and equipment or did so with five or more errors.	
Introduction to Patient	Student appropriately introduced self to the patient with one or less errors.	Student appropriately introduced self to the patient with two errors.	Student appropriately introduced self to the patient with three to four errors.	Student failed to appropriately introduce self to the patient or did so with five or more errors.	
Obtained Intake Information	Student appropriately obtained patient intake information with one or less errors.	Student appropriately obtained patient intake information with two errors.	Student appropriately obtained patient intake information with three to four errors.	Student failed to appropriately obtain patient intake information or did so with five or more errors.	
Obtained Consent	Student appropriately obtained patient consent with one or less errors.	Student appropriately obtained patient consent with two errors.	Student appropriately obtained patient consent with three to four errors.	Student failed to appropriately obtain patient consent or did so with five or more errors.	
Patient Assessment	Student performed a full patient assessment with one to two errors.	Student performed a full patient assessment with two to three errors or omitted one skill assessment.	Student performed a full patient assessment with four to five errors or omitted two skill assessments.	Student performed a full patient assessment with six or more errors or omitted three or more skills.	
Explanation of X-Ray Procedure	Student appropriately explained the X-ray procedure with no errors.	Student appropriately explained the X-ray procedure with one error.	Student appropriately explained the X-ray procedure with two to three errors.	Student failed to explain the X-ray procedure or did so with four or more errors.	
Role-Play and Written Response to Question 9	Student responded appropriately to the role-play and question 9 with no errors.	Student responded appropriately to the role-play and question 9 with one error.	Student responded appropriately to the role-play and question 9 with two to three errors.	Student failed to respond appropriately to the role-play and/or question 9 or did so with four or more errors.	

Criteria				
Assisting the Physician with Cast Application	Student appropriately assisted the physician as required with one or less errors.	Student appropriately assisted the physician as required with two errors.	Student appropriately assisted the physician as required with three to four errors.	Student failed to appropriately assist the physician as required or did so with five or more errors.
Measuring for and Explaining the Use of Crutches and the Explanation of Cast Care	Student appropriately performed the tasks with one or less errors.	Student appropriately performed the tasks with two errors.	Student appropriately performed the tasks with three to four errors.	Student failed to appropriately perform the tasks or did so with five or more errors.
Preparation and Administering of Injection	Student appropriately prepared and performed the injection with one or less errors.	Student appropriately prepared and performed the injection with two errors.	Student appropriately prepared and performed the injection with three to four errors.	Student failed to appropriately prepare and perform the injection or did so with five or more errors.
Prepare Prescription	Student appropriately performed the tasks with one or less errors.	Student appropriately performed the tasks with two errors.	Student appropriately performed the tasks with three to four errors.	Student failed to appropriately perform the tasks or did so with five or more errors.
Schedule Appointment and Provide Patient with Information	Student appropriately performed the tasks with one or less errors.	Student appropriately performed the tasks with two errors.	Student appropriately performed the tasks with three to four errors.	Student failed to appropriately perform the tasks or did so with five or more errors.
Documentation	Student properly documented all procedures with one or less errors.	Student properly documented all procedures with two errors or omitted documentation of one procedure.	Student properly documented all procedures with three to four errors or omitted documentation of two procedures.	Student properly documented all procedures with five or more errors or omitted documentation of three or more procedures.
				TOTAL

Based on the above criteria the student's grade for this assignment is: _____

(Total the points for each element scored and average for a final grade.)

Comments to the Student:

Instructor Signature: _____   Date: _____

Specialty Examination, Sigmoidoscopy

Name _____ Date _____

Elements	4 Excellent	3 Proficient	2 Adequate	1 Needs Improvement	Points
Medical Asepsis and Standard Precautions	Student correctly performed medical aseptic techniques and observed all required standard precautions with one or less errors.	Student correctly performed medical aseptic techniques and observed all required standard precautions with two errors.	Student correctly performed medical aseptic techniques and observed all required standard precautions with three to four errors.	Student failed to correctly perform medical aseptic techniques and observe all required standard precautions or did so with five or more errors.	
Supplies and Equipment	Student obtained and had available appropriate supplies and equipment with one or less errors.	Student obtained and had available appropriate supplies and equipment with two errors.	Student obtained and had available appropriate supplies and equipment with three to four errors.	Student failed to obtain or have available appropriate supplies and equipment or did so with five or more errors.	
Preparation of Room	Student appropriately prepared the room with one or less errors.	Student appropriately prepared the room with two errors.	Student appropriately prepared the room with three errors.	Student failed to appropriately prepare the room or did so with four or more errors.	
Introduction to Patient	Student appropriately introduced self to the patient with one or less errors.	Student appropriately introduced self to the patient with two errors.	Student appropriately introduced self to the patient with three to four errors.	Student failed to appropriately introduce self to the patient or did so with five or more errors.	
Obtained Intake Information	Student appropriately obtained patient intake information with one or less errors.	Student appropriately obtained patient intake information with two errors.	Student appropriately obtained patient intake information with three to four errors.	Student failed to appropriately obtain patient intake information or did so with five or more errors.	
Obtained Consent	Student appropriately obtained patient consent with one or less errors.	Student appropriately obtained patient consent with two errors.	Student appropriately obtained patient consent with three to four errors.	Student failed to appropriately obtain patient consent or did so with five or more errors.	
Patient Assessment	Student performed a full patient assessment with one to two errors.	Student performed a full patient assessment with two to three errors or omitted one skill assessment.	Student performed a full patient assessment with four to five errors or omitted two skill assessments.	Student performed a full patient assessment with six or more errors or omitted three or more skills.	
Process Guaiac Test	Student appropriately processed the test with one or less errors.	Student appropriately processed the test with two errors.	Student appropriately processed the test with three errors.	Student failed to appropriately process the test or did so with four or more errors.	
Explanation of Sigmoidoscopy Procedure	Student appropriately explained the procedure to the patient with one or less errors.	Student appropriately explained the procedure to the patient with two errors.	Student appropriately explained the procedure to the patient with three to four errors.	Student failed to appropriately explain the procedure to the patient or did so with five or more errors.	

Criteria				
Explanation of Disrobing, Gowning, Draping, and Positioning	Student appropriately explained how to disrobe, gown, drape, and position for the procedures with one or less errors.	Student appropriately explained how to disrobe, gown, drape, and position for the procedures with two errors.	Student appropriately explained how to disrobe, gown, drape, and position for the procedures with three to four errors.	Student failed to appropriately explain how to disrobe, gown, drape, and position for the procedures or did so with five or more errors.
Assisting the Physician with Sigmoidoscopy	Student appropriately assisted the physician as required with one or less errors.	Student appropriately assisted the physician as required with two errors.	Student appropriately assisted the physician as required with three to four errors.	Student failed to appropriately assist the physician as required or did so with five or more errors.
Label and Package Specimens for Laboratory	Student properly labeled and packaged the specimens to be sent to the laboratory with one or less errors.	Student properly labeled and packaged the specimens to be sent to the laboratory with two errors.	Student properly labeled and packaged the specimens to be sent to the laboratory with three to four errors.	Student failed to properly label and package the specimens to be sent to the laboratory or did so with five or more errors.
Explanation of a Fibrous Diet	Student appropriately explained a fibrous diet with no errors.	Student appropriately explained a fibrous diet with one error.	Student appropriately explained a fibrous diet with two errors.	Student failed to appropriately explain a fibrous diet or did so with three or more errors.
Response in Writing to Question 13	Student responded appropriately to question 13 with one or less errors.	Student responded appropriately to question 13 with two errors.	Student responded appropriately to question 13 with three to four errors.	Student failed to respond appropriately to question 13 or did so with five or more errors.
Schedule and Provide Patient with Follow-up Appointment Time	Student appropriately performed these tasks with one or less errors.	Student appropriately performed these tasks with two errors.	Student appropriately performed these tasks with three errors.	Student failed to appropriately perform these tasks or did so with four or more errors.
Documentation	Student properly documented all procedures with one or less errors.	Student properly documented all procedures with two errors or omitted documentation of one procedure.	Student properly documented all procedures with three to four errors or omitted documentation of two procedures.	Student properly documented all procedures with five or more errors or omitted documentation of three or more procedures.
				TOTAL

Based on the above criteria the student's grade for this assignment is: _____

(Total the points for each element scored and average for a final grade.)

Comments to the Student:

Instructor Signature: _____ Date: _____

Name _____ Date _____

CASE STUDY 59   *Endocrine Disorder*

Elements	4 Excellent	3 Proficient	2 Adequate	1 Needs Improvement	Points
New Patient Chart	Student correctly created a new patient chart electronically and identified the forms requiring a patient signature with one or less errors.	Student correctly created a new patient chart electronically and identified the forms requiring a patient signature with two errors.	Student correctly created a new patient chart electronically and identified the forms requiring a patient signature with three to four errors.	Student failed to correctly create a new patient chart electronically and identify the forms requiring a patient signature or did so with five or more errors.	
Medical Asepsis and Standard Precautions	Student correctly performed medical aseptic techniques and observed all required standard precautions with one or less errors.	Student correctly performed medical aseptic techniques and observed all required standard precautions with two errors.	Student correctly performed medical aseptic techniques and observed all required standard precautions with three to four errors.	Student failed to correctly perform medical aseptic techniques and observe all required standard precautions or did so with five or more errors.	
Supplies and Equipment	Student obtained and had available appropriate supplies and equipment with one or less errors.	Student obtained and had available appropriate supplies and equipment with two errors.	Student obtained and had available appropriate supplies and equipment with three to four errors.	Student failed to obtain or have available appropriate supplies and equipment or did so with five or more errors.	
Response to Question 3	Student correctly identified the equipment and supplies needed for the procedures with one or less errors.	Student correctly identified the equipment and supplies needed for the procedures with two errors.	Student correctly identified the equipment and supplies needed for the procedures with three to four errors.	Student correctly identified the equipment and supplies needed for the procedures with five or more errors or failed to identify the equipment and supplies needed for the procedures.	
Introduction to Patient	Student appropriately introduced self to the patient with one or less errors.	Student appropriately introduced self to the patient with two errors.	Student appropriately introduced self to the patient with three to four errors.	Student failed to appropriately introduce self to the patient or did so with five or more errors.	
Obtained Intake Information	Student appropriately obtained patient intake information with one or less errors.	Student appropriately obtained patient intake information with two errors.	Student appropriately obtained patient intake information with three to four errors.	Student failed to appropriately obtain patient intake information or did so with five or more errors.	
Obtained Consent	Student appropriately obtained patient consent with one or less errors.	Student appropriately obtained patient consent with two errors.	Student appropriately obtained patient consent with three to four errors.	Student failed to appropriately obtain patient consent or did so with five or more errors.	

Skill				
Patient Assessment • Height • Weight • Temperature • Pulse • Respiration • Blood Pressure	Student performed a full patient assessment with one to two errors.	Student performed a full patient assessment with two to three errors or omitted one skill assessment.	Student performed a full patient assessment with four to five errors or omitted two skill assessments.	Student performed a full patient assessment with six or more errors or omitted three or more skills.
Patient Instructions on Obtaining a Clean-Catch Urine Sample	Student provided appropriate patient instruction with one or less errors.	Student provided appropriate patient instruction with two errors.	Student provided appropriate patient instruction with three to four errors.	Student failed to provide appropriate patient instruction or did so with five or more errors.
Perform Pregnancy Test and a UA Physical and Chemical Examination	Student performed the tests with no errors.	Student performed the tests with one error.	Student performed the tests with two errors.	Student performed the tests with three or more errors.
Explanation of Prenatal Examination	Student appropriately explained the examination to the patient with one or less errors.	Student appropriately explained the examination to the patient with two errors.	Student appropriately explained the examination to the patient with three to four errors.	Student failed to appropriately explain the examination to the patient or did so with five or more errors.
Explanation of Disrobing, Gowning, and Draping	Student appropriately explained how to disrobe, gown, and drape for the procedures with one or less errors.	Student appropriately explained how to disrobe, gown, and drape for the procedures with two errors.	Student appropriately explained how to disrobe, gown, and drape for the procedures with three to four errors.	Student failed to appropriately explain how to disrobe, gown, and drape for the procedures or did so with five or more errors.
Patient Positioning	Student appropriately positioned and draped the patient for her examination with no errors.	Student appropriately positioned and draped the patient for her examination with one error.	Student appropriately positioned and draped the patient for her examination with two errors.	Student failed to appropriately position and drape the patient for her examination or did so with three or more errors.
Assisting the Physician with the Prenatal Examination	Student appropriately assisted the physician as required with one or less errors.	Student appropriately assisted the physician as required with two errors.	Student appropriately assisted the physician as required with three to four errors.	Student failed to appropriately assist the physician as required or did so with five or more errors.
Perform Venipuncture	Student properly performed a venipuncture with one or less errors.	Student properly performed a venipuncture with two errors.	Student properly performed a venipuncture with three to four errors.	Student failed to properly perform a venipuncture or did so with five or more errors.
Identifying Number and Color of Tubes Needed	Student correctly identified the appropriate number of tubes and the appropriate color of tubes for the tests requested with one or less errors.	Student correctly identified the appropriate number of tubes and the appropriate color of tubes for the tests requested with two errors.	Student correctly identified the appropriate number of tubes and the appropriate color of tubes for the tests requested with three to four errors.	Student failed to correctly identify the appropriate number of tubes and the appropriate color of tubes for the tests requested or did so with five or more errors.

	Student answered the question properly with one or less errors.	Student answered the question properly with two errors.	Student answered the question properly with three errors.	Student failed to answer the question properly or did so with four or more errors.	
Response to Question 18	Student answered the question properly with one or less errors.	Student answered the question properly with two errors.	Student answered the question properly with three errors.	Student failed to answer the question properly or did so with four or more errors.	
Package Specimens for Laboratory	Student properly packaged the specimens to be sent to the laboratory with one or less errors.	Student properly packaged the specimens to be sent to the laboratory with two errors.	Student properly packaged the specimens to be sent to the laboratory with three to four errors.	Student failed to properly package the specimens to be sent to the laboratory or did so with five or more errors.	
Response to Question 21	Student answered the question properly with one or less errors.	Student answered the question properly with two errors.	Student answered the question properly with three errors.	Student failed to answer the question properly or did so with four or more errors.	
Documentation	Student properly documented all procedures with one or less errors.	Student properly documented all procedures with two errors or omitted documentation of one procedure.	Student properly documented all procedures with three to four errors or omitted documentation of two procedures.	Student properly documented all procedures with five or more errors or omitted documentation of two or more procedures.	
					TOTAL

Based on the above criteria the student's grade for this assignment is: _____

(Total the points for each element scored and average for a final grade.)

Comments to the Student:

Instructor Signature: _____   Date: _____

Prescription Drug Abuse, Patient Advocate

Name _____ Date _____

Elements	4 Excellent	3 Proficient	2 Adequate	1 Needs Improvement	Points
Medical Asepsis and Standard Precautions	Student correctly performed medical aseptic techniques and observed all required standard precautions with one or less errors.	Student correctly performed medical aseptic techniques and observed all required standard precautions with two errors.	Student correctly performed medical aseptic techniques and observed all required standard precautions with three to four errors.	Student failed to correctly perform medical aseptic techniques and observe all required standard precautions or did so with five or more errors.	
Introduction to Patient	Student appropriately introduced self to the patient with one or less errors.	Student appropriately introduced self to the patient with two errors.	Student appropriately introduced self to the patient with three to four errors.	Student failed to appropriately introduce self to the patient or did so with five or more errors.	
Obtained Intake Information	Student appropriately obtained patient intake information with one or less errors.	Student appropriately obtained patient intake information with two errors.	Student appropriately obtained patient intake information with three to four errors.	Student failed to appropriately obtain patient intake information or did so with five or more errors.	
Patient Assessment • Height • Weight • Temperature • Pulse • Respiration • Blood Pressure	Student performed a full patient assessment with one to two errors.	Student performed a full patient assessment with two to three errors or omitted one skill assessment.	Student performed a full patient assessment with four to five errors or omitted two skill assessments.	Student performed a full patient assessment with six or more errors or omitted three or more skills.	
Patient Instructions	Student provided appropriate patient instruction with one or less errors.	Student provided appropriate patient instruction with two errors.	Student provided appropriate patient instruction with three to four errors.	Student failed to provide appropriate patient instructions or did so with five or more errors.	
Response to Question 6	Student responded appropriately to question 6.	N/A	N/A	Student failed to respond to question 6 or did so inappropriately.	
Response to Question 7	Student responded appropriately to question 7 with no errors.	Student responded appropriately to question 7 with one error.	Student responded appropriately to question 7 with two errors.	Student failed to respond appropriately to question 7 or did so with three or more errors.	
Response to Question 8	Student responded appropriately to question 8.	N/A	N/A	Student failed to respond to question 8 or did so inappropriately.	

Response to Question 9	Student responded appropriately to question 9 with no errors.	Student responded appropriately to question 9 with one error.	Student responded appropriately to question 9 with two errors.	Student failed to respond appropriately to question 9 or did so with three or more errors.	
Role-Play Patient Advocacy	Student demonstrated the ability to act as a patient advocate with one or less errors.	Student demonstrated the ability to act as a patient advocate with two errors.	Student demonstrated the ability to act as a patient advocate with three errors.	Student failed to demonstrate the ability to act as a patient advocate or did so with four or more errors.	
Patient Pamphlet	Student created a patient pamphlet with one or less errors.	Student created a patient pamphlet with two errors.	Student created a patient pamphlet with three errors.	Student failed to create a patient pamphlet or did so with four or more errors.	
				TOTAL	

Based on the above criteria the student's grade for this assignment is: _____

(Total the points for each element scored and average for a final grade.)

Comments to the Student:

Instructor Signature: _____   Date: _____

298

CASE STUDY 61 *Possible Spousal Abuse Emergency Triage*

Name _____ Date _____

Elements	4 Excellent	3 Proficient	2 Adequate	1 Needs Improvement	Points
Patient Greeting	Student appropriately greeted the patient.	N/A	N/A	Student failed to appropriately greet the patient.	
Evaluating for Effectiveness	Student employed observational and active listening skills and provided appropriate feedback with one or less errors.	Student employed observational and active listening skills and provided appropriate feedback with two errors.	Student employed observational and active listening skills and provided appropriate feedback with three to four errors.	Student failed to employ observational and active listening skills and provide appropriate feedback or did so with five or more errors.	
Recognizing and Responding to an Emergency Walk-In Patient	Student appropriately recognized and responded to an emergency walk-in patient with no errors.	Student appropriately recognized and responded to an emergency walk-in patient with one error.	Student appropriately recognized and responded to an emergency walk-in patient with two to three errors.	Student failed to appropriately recognize and respond to an emergency walk-in patient or did so with four or more errors.	
Communication with Distraught Patient	Student demonstrated the ability to professionally communicate with a distraught patient.	N/A	N/A	Student failed to professionally communicate with a distraught patient.	
Communicating with an Angry Spouse	Student demonstrated the ability to professionally communicate with an angry spouse.	N/A	N/A	Student failed to professionally communicate with an angry spouse.	
Response to Question 2	Student appropriately responded and defended his or her responses to the questions.	Student appropriately responded to the questions but failed to defend his or her responses.	Student inappropriately responded and defended his or her response to the questions.	Student failed to respond or defend the questions.	
Response to Question 3	Student appropriately responded and defended his or her response.	Student appropriately responded but failed to defend his or her response.	Student inappropriately responded and defended his or her response to the question.	Student failed to respond or defend the question.	
Response to Question 4	Student correctly identified the verbal and nonverbal communication that occurred between the couple.	N/A	N/A	Student failed to identify the verbal and nonverbal communication that occurred between the couple.	
Response to Question 5	Student identified the appropriate communication skills needed for this type of situation.	N/A	N/A	Student failed to identify the appropriate communication skills needed for this situation.	

		N/A	N/A
Response to Question 7	Student appropriately defended his or her actions in the scenario and described what may happen next.	N/A	Student failed to defend his or her actions in the scenario and describe what may happen next.
Response to Question 8 One-Page Paper	Student responded to the questions with a one-page paper with one or less errors.	Student responded to the questions with a one-page paper with two errors.	Student responded to the questions with a one-page paper with three to four errors.	Student failed to submit a paper or did so with five or more errors.
				TOTAL

Based on the above criteria the student's grade for this assignment is: _____

(Total the points for each element scored and average for a final grade.)

Comments to the Student:

Instructor Signature: _____   Date: _____

Walk-In, Triage, and Follow-Up

Name _____ Date _____

Elements	4 Excellent	3 Proficient	2 Adequate	1 Needs Improvement	Points
Introduction to Patient	Student appropriately introduced self to the patient with one or less errors.	Student appropriately introduced self to the patient with two errors.	Student appropriately introduced self to the patient with three to four errors.	Student failed to appropriately introduce self to the patient or did so with five or more errors.	
Medical Asepsis and Standard Precautions	Student correctly performed medical aseptic techniques and observed all required standard precautions with one or less errors.	Student correctly performed medical aseptic techniques and observed all required standard precautions with two errors.	Student correctly performed medical aseptic techniques and observed all required standard precautions with three to four errors.	Student failed to correctly perform medical aseptic techniques and observe all required standard precautions or did so with five or more errors.	
Obtained Consent	Student appropriately obtained patient consent with one or less errors.	Student appropriately obtained patient consent with two errors.	Student appropriately obtained patient consent with three to four errors.	Student failed to appropriately obtain patient consent or did so with five or more errors.	
Patient Assessment • Height • Weight • Temperature • Pulse • Respiration • Blood Pressure	Student performed a full patient assessment with one to two errors.	Student performed a full patient assessment with two to three errors or omitted one skill assessment.	Student performed a full patient assessment with four to five errors or omitted two skill assessments.	Student performed a full patient assessment with six or more errors or omitted three or more skills.	
Evaluating for Effectiveness	Student employed observational and active listening skills and provided appropriate feedback with one or less errors.	Student employed observational and active listening skills and provided appropriate feedback with two errors.	Student employed observational and active listening skills and provided appropriate feedback with three to four errors.	Student failed to employ observational and active listening skills and provide appropriate feedback or did so with five or more errors.	
Patient Interviewing Techniques	Student effectively used exploratory, open-ended, and direct questions when interviewing the patient and submitted a written overview of the interview.	Student effectively used exploratory, open-ended, and direct questions when interviewing the patient but failed to submit a written overview.	Student failed to effectively interview the patient using the different types of questions but submitted a written overview of his or her interview.	Student failed to use different types of questions to effectively interview the patient and failed to submit a written overview of his or her interview.	
Explanation of Disrobing, Gowning, and Draping	Student appropriately explained how to disrobe, gown, and drape for the procedures with one or less errors.	Student appropriately explained how to disrobe, gown, and drape for the procedures with two errors.	Student appropriately explained how to disrobe, gown, and drape for the procedures with three to four errors.	Student failed to appropriately explain how to disrobe, gown, and drape for the procedures or did so with five or more errors.	

Assisting the Physician	Student appropriately assisted the physician as required with one or less errors.	Student appropriately assisted the physician as required with two errors.	Student appropriately assisted the physician as required with three to four errors.	Student appropriately assisted the physician as required or did so with five or more errors.
Explanation of X-Ray Procedure	Student appropriately explained the X-ray procedure with no errors.	Student appropriately explained the X-ray procedure with one error.	Student appropriately explained the X-ray procedure with two to three errors.	Student failed to explain the X-ray procedure or did so with four or more errors.
Notifying Emergency Services	Student notified Emergency Services and provided them with correct information while maintaining professional communication and behavior.	N/A	N/A	Student failed to notify Emergency Services or notified Emergency Services maintaining professional communication techniques and omitted relevant information or notified Emergency Services and provided them with the correct information without demonstrating appropriate professional communication and behavior.
Question 10 Patient Advocate	Student appropriately described the role of a patient advocate.	N/A	N/A	Student failed to appropriately describe the role of a patient advocate.
Documentation	Student properly documented all procedures with one or less errors.	Student properly documented all procedures with two errors or omitted documentation of one procedure.	Student properly documented all procedures with three to four errors or omitted documentation of two procedures.	Student properly documented all procedures with five or more errors or omitted documentation of three or more procedures.
Responding to Emergency Walk-In Patient	Student appropriately responded to an emergency walk-in patient with no errors.	Student appropriately responded to an emergency walk-in patient with one error.	Student appropriately responded to an emergency walk-in patient with two to three errors.	Student failed to appropriately respond to an emergency walk-in patient or did so with four or more errors.
				TOTAL

Based on the above criteria the student's grade for this assignment is: _____

(Total the points for each element scored and average for a final grade.)

Comments to the Student:

Instructor Signature: _____   Date: _____

CASE STUDY 63 *Type 1 Diabetes, Laboratory Tests*

Name _____ Date _____

Elements	4 Excellent	3 Proficient	2 Adequate	1 Needs Improvement	Points
Medical Asepsis and Standard Precautions	Student correctly performed medical aseptic techniques and observed all required standard precautions with one or less errors.	Student correctly performed medical aseptic techniques and observed all required standard precautions with two errors.	Student correctly performed medical aseptic techniques and observed all required standard precautions with three to four errors.	Student failed to correctly perform medical aseptic techniques and observe all required standard precautions or did so with five or more errors.	
Supplies and Equipment	Student obtained and had available appropriate supplies and equipment with one or less errors.	Student obtained and had available appropriate supplies and equipment with two errors.	Student obtained and had available appropriate supplies and equipment with three to four errors.	Student failed to obtain or have available appropriate supplies and equipment or did so with five or more errors.	
Introduction to Patient	Student appropriately introduced self to the patient with one or less errors.	Student appropriately introduced self to the patient with two errors.	Student appropriately introduced self to the patient with three to four errors.	Student failed to appropriately introduce self to the patient or did so with five or more errors.	
Obtained Intake Information	Student appropriately obtained patient intake information with one or less errors.	Student appropriately obtained patient intake information with two errors.	Student appropriately obtained patient intake information with three to four errors.	Student failed to appropriately obtain patient intake information or did so with five or more errors.	
Explanation of Procedure(s)	Student appropriately explained the procedure(s) to the patient with one or less errors.	Student appropriately explained the procedure(s) to the patient with two errors.	Student appropriately explained the procedure(s) to the patient with three to four errors.	Student failed to appropriately explain the procedure(s) to the patient or did so with five or more errors.	
Obtained Consent	Student appropriately obtained patient consent with one or less errors.	Student appropriately obtained patient consent with two errors.	Student appropriately obtained patient consent with three to four errors.	Student failed to appropriately obtain patient consent or did so with five or more errors.	
Patient Assessment • **Height** • **Weight** • **Temperature** • **Pulse** • **Respiration** • **Blood Pressure**	Student performed a full patient assessment with one to two errors.	Student performed a full patient assessment with two to three errors or omitted one skill assessment.	Student performed a full patient assessment with four to five errors or omitted two skill assessments.	Student performed a full patient assessment with six or more errors or omitted three or more skills.	
Patient Instructions	Student provided appropriate patient instruction with one or less errors.	Student provided appropriate patient instruction with two errors.	Student provided appropriate patient instruction with three to four errors.	Student failed to provide appropriate patient instruction or did so with five or more errors.	

	Student properly performed a UA dip with no errors.	Student properly performed a UA dip with one error.	Student properly performed a UA dip with two to three errors.	Student failed to properly perform a UA dip or did so with five or more errors.
Perform UA Dip	Student properly performed a UA dip with no errors.	Student properly performed a UA dip with one error.	Student properly performed a UA dip with two to three errors.	Student failed to properly perform a UA dip or did so with five or more errors.
Capillary Puncture	Student properly performed a capillary puncture with one or less errors.	Student properly performed a capillary puncture with two errors.	Student properly performed a capillary puncture with three to four errors.	Student failed to properly perform a capillary puncture or did so with five or more errors.
Perform POCT Blood Glucose	Student properly performed a POCT blood glucose with no errors.	Student properly performed a POCT blood glucose with two errors.	Student properly performed a POCT blood glucose with two to three errors.	Student failed to properly perform a POCT blood glucose or did so with five or more errors.
Explanation of Preparation for Three-Hour FBS	Student appropriately explained the preparation for a three-hour FBS to the patient with one or less errors.	Student appropriately explained the preparation for a three-hour FBS to the patient with two errors.	Student appropriately explained the preparation for a three-hour FBS to the patient with three to four errors.	Student failed to appropriately explain the preparation for a three-hour FBS to the patient or did so with five or more errors.
Perform Venipuncture 1	Student properly performed a venipuncture with one or less errors.	Student properly performed a venipuncture with two errors.	Student properly performed a venipuncture with three to four errors.	Student failed to properly perform a venipuncture or did so with five or more errors.
Perform Venipuncture 2	Student properly performed a venipuncture with one or less errors.	Student properly performed a venipuncture with two errors.	Student properly performed a venipuncture with three to four errors.	Student failed to properly perform a venipuncture or did so with five or more errors.
Timing of Venipunctures	Student performed the second venipuncture 45 minutes after the first venipuncture, allowing for classroom environment.	N/A	N/A	Student failed to perform the second venipuncture 45 minutes after the first venipuncture, allowing for classroom environment.
HbA1C	Student properly performed an HbA1C with one or less errors.	Student properly performed an HbA1C with two errors.	Student properly performed an HbA1C with three to four errors.	Student failed to properly perform an HbA1C or did so with five or more errors.
Response to Question 13	Student appropriately responded to the question.	N/A	N/A	Student failed to appropriately respond to the question.
Response to Question 14	Student appropriately responded to the question.	N/A	N/A	Student failed to appropriately respond to the question.
Response to Question 15	Student appropriately responded to the question.	N/A	N/A	Student failed to appropriately respond to the question.
Response to Question 16	Student appropriately responded to the question.	N/A	N/A	Student failed to appropriately respond to the question.

Schedule GTT	Student properly scheduled a GTT with one or less errors.	Student properly scheduled a GTT with two errors.	Student properly scheduled a GTT with three to four errors.	Student failed to properly schedule a GTT or did so with five or more errors.
Documentation	Student properly documented all procedures with one or less errors.	Student properly documented all procedures with two errors or omitted documentation of one procedure.	Student properly documented all procedures with three to four errors or omitted documentation of two procedures.	Student properly documented all procedures with five or more errors or omitted documentation of three or more procedures.
				TOTAL

Based on the above criteria the student's grade for this assignment is: _____

(Total the points for each element scored and average for a final grade.)

Comments to the Student:

Instructor Signature: _____   Date: _____

Insurance Billing and Coding, Laboratory Tests

Name _____ Date _____

Elements	4 Excellent	3 Proficient	2 Adequate	1 Needs Improvement	Points
Diagnosis	Student correctly identified the diagnosis.	N/A	N/A	Student failed to correctly identify the diagnosis.	
Services Provided	Student correctly identified all services provided with one or less errors.	Student correctly identified all services provided with two errors.	Student correctly identified all services provided with three to four errors.	Student failed to correctly identify all services provided or did so with five or more errors.	
ICD-9-CM Code	Student correctly identified the diagnosis code.	N/A	N/A	Student failed to correctly identify the diagnosis code.	
CPT Codes	Student correctly identified the required CPT codes with one or less errors.	Student correctly identified the required CPT codes with two errors.	Student correctly identified the required CPT codes with three to four errors.	Student failed to correctly identify the required CPT codes or did so with five or more errors.	
Insurance Claim Form	Student appropriately completed an insurance claim form with one or less errors.	Student appropriately completed an insurance claim form with two errors.	Student appropriately completed an insurance claim form with three to four errors.	Student failed to appropriately complete an insurance claim form or did so with five or more errors.	
				TOTAL	

Based on the above criteria the student's grade for this assignment is: _____

(Total the points for each element scored and average for a final grade.)

Comments to the Student:

Instructor Signature: _____ Date: _____

Patient Education, Injections, Dosage Calculation

Name _____ Date _____

Elements	4 Excellent	3 Proficient	2 Adequate	1 Needs Improvement	Points
Medical Asepsis and Standard Precautions	Student correctly performed medical aseptic techniques and observed all required standard precautions with one or less errors.	Student correctly performed medical aseptic techniques and observed all required standard precautions with two errors.	Student correctly performed medical aseptic techniques and observed all precautions with three to four errors.	Student failed to correctly perform medical aseptic techniques and observe all required standard precautions or did so with five or more errors.	
Supplies and Equipment	Student obtained and had available appropriate supplies and equipment with one or less errors.	Student obtained and had available appropriate supplies and equipment with two errors.	Student obtained and had available appropriate supplies and equipment with three to four errors.	Student failed to obtain or have available appropriate supplies and equipment or did so with five or more errors.	
Introduction to Patient	Student appropriately introduced self to the patient with one or less errors.	Student appropriately introduced self to the patient with two errors.	Student appropriately introduced self to the patient with three to four errors.	Student failed to appropriately introduce self to the patient or did so with five or more errors.	
Obtained Intake Information	Student appropriately obtained patient intake information with one or less errors.	Student appropriately obtained patient intake information with two errors.	Student appropriately obtained patient intake information with three to four errors.	Student failed to appropriately obtain patient intake information or did so with five or more errors.	
Explanation of Procedure(s)	Student appropriately explained the procedure(s) to the patient, including the risks and side effects, with one or less errors.	Student appropriately explained the procedure(s) to the patient, including the risks and side effects, with two errors.	Student appropriately explained the procedure(s) to the patient, including the risks and side effects with three to four errors.	Student failed to appropriately explain the procedure(s) to the patient, including the risks and side effects, or did so with five or more errors.	
Obtained Consent	Student appropriately obtained patient consent with one or less errors.	Student appropriately obtained patient consent with two errors.	Student appropriately obtained patient consent with three to four errors.	Student failed to appropriately obtain patient consent or did so with five or more errors.	
Patient Assessment • Height • Weight • Temperature • Pulse • Respiration • Blood Pressure	Student performed a full patient assessment with one to two errors.	Student performed a full patient assessment with two to three errors or omitted one skill assessment.	Student performed a full patient assessment with four to five errors or omitted two skill assessments.	Student performed a full patient assessment with six or more errors or omitted three or more skills.	
Patient Instructions	Student provided appropriate patient instruction with one or less errors.	Student provided appropriate patient instruction with two errors.	Student provided appropriate patient instruction with three to four errors.	Student failed to provide appropriate patient instruction or did so with five or more errors.	

	Student properly performed the injection with one or less errors.	Student properly performed the injection with two errors.	Student properly performed the injection with three errors.	Student failed to properly perform the injection or did so with four or more errors.	
Injection	Student properly performed the injection with one or less errors.	Student properly performed the injection with two errors.	Student properly performed the injection with three errors.	Student failed to properly perform the injection or did so with four or more errors.	
Response to Question 9	Student appropriately responded to the question.	N/A	N/A	Student failed to appropriately respond to the question.	
Demonstration and Patient Education	Student properly demonstrated and provided appropriate patient education instructions with one or less errors.	Student properly demonstrated and provided appropriate patient education instructions with two errors.	Student properly demonstrated and provided appropriate patient education instructions with three errors.	Student failed to properly demonstrate and provide appropriate patient education instructions or did so with four or more errors.	
Documentation	Student properly documented all procedures with one or less errors.	Student properly documented all procedures with two errors or omitted documentation of one procedure.	Student properly documented all procedures with three to four errors or omitted documentation of two procedures.	Student properly documented all procedures with five or more errors or omitted documentation of three or more procedures.	
				TOTAL	

Based on the above criteria the student's grade for this assignment is: _____

(Total the points for each element scored and average for a final grade.)

Comments to the Student:

Instructor Signature: _____   Date: _____

First Aid–Seizures

Name _____ Date _____

Elements	4 Excellent	3 Proficient	2 Adequate	1 Needs Improvement	Points
Response to Question 1	Student responded appropriately to question 1.	N/A	N/A	Student failed to respond to question 1 or did so inappropriately.	
Response to Question 2	Student submitted a list of equipment and supplies.	N/A	N/A	Student failed to submit a list of equipment and supplies.	
Response to Question 3	Student submitted a paper regarding patient care during a grand mal seizure.	N/A	N/A	Student failed to submit a paper regarding patient care during a grand mal seizure.	
Patient Greeting	Student appropriately greeted the patient.	N/A	N/A	Student failed to appropriately greet the patient.	
Explanation of Physician Unavailability	Student addressed physician unavailability during the role-play.	N/A	N/A	Student failed to address physician unavailability during the role-play.	
Communication with Anxious Patient	Student demonstrated the ability to professionally communicate with an anxious patient.	N/A	N/A	Student failed to demonstrate the ability to professionally communicate with an anxious patient.	
Responding to Emergency	Student appropriately responded to an emergency with no errors.	Student appropriately responded to an emergency with one error.	Student appropriately responded to an emergency with two to three errors.	Student failed to appropriately respond to an emergency or did so with four or more errors.	
Notifying Emergency Services	Student notified Emergency Services and provided them with correct information while maintaining professional communication and behavior.	N/A	N/A	Student failed to notify Emergency Services or notified Emergency Services while maintaining professional communication techniques and omitted relevant information or notified Emergency Services and provided them with the correct information without demonstrating appropriate professional communication and behavior.	
Assessment and Triage	Student accurately assessed and triaged the patient with one or less errors.	Student accurately assessed and triaged the patient with two errors.	Student accurately assessed and triaged the patient with three four errors.	Student failed to accurately assess and triage the patient or did so with five or more errors.	

Patient Assessment • **Temperature** • **Pulse** • **Respiration** • **Blood Pressure**	Student performed a patient assessment with one or less errors.	Student performed a patient assessment with two errors.	Student performed a patient assessment with three errors.	Student failed to perform a patient assessment or did so with four or more errors.
Medical Asepsis and Standard Precautions	Student correctly performed medical aseptic techniques and observed all required standard precautions with one or less errors.	Student correctly performed medical aseptic techniques and observed all required standard precautions with two errors.	Student correctly performed medical aseptic techniques and observed all required standard precautions with three to four errors.	Student failed to correctly perform medical aseptic techniques and observe all required standard precautions or did so with five or more errors.
Assisting the Physician	Student appropriately assisted the physician as required with one or less errors.	Student appropriately assisted the physician as required with two errors.	Student appropriately assisted the physician as required with three to four errors.	Student failed to appropriately assist the physician as required or did so with five or more errors.
Evaluating for Effectiveness	Student employed observational and active listening skills and provided appropriate feedback with one or less errors.	Student employed observational and active listening skills and provided appropriate feedback with two errors.	Student employed observational and active listening skills and provided appropriate feedback with three to four errors.	Student failed to employ observational and active listening skills and provide appropriate feedback or did so with five or more errors.
Hook Up and Starting Oxygen	Student correctly hooked up and started the patient on oxygen at the correct rate with one or less errors.	Student correctly hooked up and started the patient on oxygen at the correct rate with two errors.	Student correctly hooked up and started the patient on oxygen at the correct rate with three to four errors.	Student failed to correctly hook up and start the patient on oxygen at the correct rate or did so with five or more errors.
Pulse Oximetry	Student attached the pulse oximetry to the patient.	N/A	N/A	Student failed to attach the pulse oximetry to the patient.
IV Tubing and Catheter	Student correctly set up the IV tubing and catheter with no errors.	Student correctly set up the IV tubing and catheter with one error.	Student correctly set up the IV tubing and catheter with two errors.	Student failed to correctly set up the IV tubing and catheter or did so with three or more errors.
Drawing Medication	Student correctly drew the prescribed medication with no errors.	N/A	Student correctly drew the prescribed medication with one or more errors.	Student failed to correctly draw the prescribed medication.
Capillary Blood Draw	Student performed a finger stick on the patient with no errors.	Student performed a finger stick on the patient with one error.	Student performed a finger stick on the patient with two errors.	Student failed to perform a finger stick or did so with three or more errors.
Glucose Test	Student correctly performed a blood sugar test with no errors.	N/A	N/A	Student failed to correctly perform a glucose test or did so with one or more errors.
Response to Question 7	Student responded appropriately to question 7.	N/A	N/A	Student failed to respond to question 7 or did so inappropriately.
Prepare ECG Machine	Student correctly prepared the ECG machine with no errors.	N/A	Student correctly prepared the ECG machine with one error.	Student failed to correctly prepare the ECG machine or did so with two or more errors.

Criteria				
Donning Gloves for Cleaning Vomit	Student donned gloves before cleaning vomit.	N/A	N/A	Student failed to don gloves before cleaning vomit.
Properly Dispose of Waste Materials	Student properly disposed of waste materials.	N/A	N/A	Student failed to properly dispose of waste materials.
Response to Question 11	Student responded appropriately to question 11 with one or less errors.	Student responded appropriately to question 11 with two errors.	Student responded appropriately to question 11 with three errors.	Student failed to respond appropriately to question 11 or did so with four or more errors.
Documentation	Student properly documented all procedures with one or less errors.	Student properly documented all procedures with two errors or omitted documentation of one procedure.	Student properly documented all procedures with three to four errors or omitted documentation of two procedures.	Student properly documented all procedures with five or more errors or omitted documentation of three or more procedures.
Response to Question 13	Student provided a well-thought-out response to the questions in question 13.	N/A	N/A	Student failed to provide a well-thought-out response to the questions in question 13.
				TOTAL

Based on the above criteria the student's grade for this assignment is: _____

(Total the points for each element scored and average for a final grade.)

Comments to the Student:

Instructor Signature: _____ Date: _____

313

Patient Termination

Name _____ Date _____

Elements	4 Excellent	3 Proficient	2 Adequate	1 Needs Improvement	Points
Role-Play Scenario 1	Student participated in the role-play scenario.	N/A	N/A	Student failed to participate in the role-play scenario.	
Internet Search	Student correctly performed an Internet search and located updated requirements for patient termination within the last six months with one or less errors.	Student correctly performed an Internet search and located updated requirements for patient termination within the last six months with two errors.	Student correctly performed an Internet search and located updated requirements for patient termination within the last six months with three errors.	Student failed to correctly perform an Internet search or did not locate relevant information dated within the last six months or did so with four or more errors.	
Document for Policy and Procedure Manual	Student compiled information into a professional document with one or less errors.	Student compiled information into a professional document with two errors.	Student compiled information into a professional document with three errors.	Student failed to compile information into a professional document or did so with four or more errors.	
Watermark	Student correctly placed a watermark into the document.	N/A	N/A	Student failed to correctly place a watermark into the document.	
Fundamental Writing Skills	Student appropriately used medical terminology, sentence structure, grammar, and punctuation with one or less errors.	Student appropriately used medical terminology, sentence structure, grammar, and punctuation with two errors.	Student appropriately used medical terminology, sentence structure, grammar, and punctuation with three to four errors.	Student failed to appropriately use medical terminology, sentence structure, grammar, and punctuation or did so with five or more errors.	
Proofreading	Student implemented the required changes in the final draft of his or her proofread document.	N/A	N/A	Student failed to implement the required changes to the final draft of his or her proofread document.	
Letter	Student correctly formatted a formal letter of notification with one or less errors.	Student correctly formatted a formal letter of notification with two errors.	Student correctly formatted a formal letter of notification with three errors.	Student failed to correctly format a formal letter of notification or did so with four or more errors.	
Fundamental Writing Skills of Letter	Student appropriately used medical terminology, sentence structure, grammar, and punctuation with one or less errors.	Student appropriately used medical terminology, sentence structure, grammar, and punctuation with two errors.	Student appropriately used medical terminology, sentence structure, grammar, and punctuation with three errors.	Student failed to appropriately use medical terminology, sentence structure, grammar, and punctuation or did so with four or more errors.	

Response to Question 6	Student correctly researched and identified the most cost-effective method for mailing the notification letter with delivery confirmation.	N/A	N/A	Student failed to correctly research and identify the most cost-effective method for mailing the notification letter with delivery confirmation.	
Response to Question 7	Student correctly explained mail classifications with no errors.	Student correctly explained mail classifications with one error.	Student correctly explained mail classifications with two to three errors.	Student failed to correctly explain mail classifications or did so with four or more errors.	
Preparing Letter and Envelope	Student correctly prepared the letter and envelope, following postal guidelines for outgoing mail, with no errors.	Student correctly prepared the letter and envelope, following postal guidelines for outgoing mail, with one error.	Student correctly prepared the letter and envelope, following postal guidelines for outgoing mail, with two errors.	Student failed to correctly prepare the letter and envelope, following postal guidelines for outgoing mail, or did so with three or more errors.	
				TOTAL	

Based on the above criteria the student's grade for this assignment is: _____

(Total the points for each element scored and average for a final grade.)

Comments to the Student:

Instructor Signature: _____   Date: _____

Job Search–Interview Administration

Name _____ Date _____

Elements	4 Excellent	3 Proficient	2 Adequate	1 Needs Improvement	Points
Create or Update a Current Resume	Student correctly created or updated a current resume with one or less errors.	Student correctly created or updated a current resume with two errors.	Student correctly created or updated a current resume with three to four errors.	Student failed to correctly create or update a current resume or did so with five or more errors.	
Locate Six Employment Positions	Student located six positions that he or she is qualified for (two in each category listed).	Student located five positions that he or she is qualified for.	Student located four positions that he or she is qualified for.	Student located under four positions that he or she is qualified for.	
Write a Cover Letter for Desired Position	Student correctly wrote a cover letter for the desired position with one or less errors.	Student correctly wrote a cover letter for the desired position with two errors.	Student correctly wrote a cover letter for the desired position with three to four errors.	Student failed to correctly write a cover letter for the desired position or did so with five or more errors.	
Request an Interview by Telephone	Student appropriately requested an interview with one or less errors.	Student appropriately requested an interview with two errors.	Student appropriately requested an interview with three to four errors.	Student failed to appropriately request an interview or did so with five or more errors.	
Interview for Position	Student appropriately interviewed for a position with one or less errors.	Student appropriately interviewed for a position with two errors.	Student appropriately interviewed for a position with three to four errors.	Student failed to appropriately interview for a position or did so with five or more errors.	
Thank-You Card Follow-up	Student developed and delivered a professional thank-you card with no errors.	N/A	N/A	Student failed to develop and deliver a professional thank-you card.	
				TOTAL	

Based on the above criteria the student's grade for this assignment is: _____
(Total the points for each element scored and average for a final grade.)

Comments to the Student:

Instructor Signature: _____ Date: _____

CASE STUDY **69** *Annual Evaluation*

Name _____ Date _____

Elements	4 Excellent	3 Proficient	2 Adequate	1 Needs Improvement	Points
Self-Evaluation	Student correctly completed the self-evaluation form within the assigned time frame with one or less errors.	Student correctly completed the self-evaluation form within the assigned time frame with two errors.	Student correctly completed the self-evaluation form within the assigned time frame with three to four errors.	Student failed to correctly complete the self-evaluation form within the assigned time frame or did so with five or more errors.	
Evaluation Interview	Student conducted self in an appropriate manner, answered questions, and provided input during the evaluation to a standard of Excellence.	Student conducted self in an appropriate manner, answered questions, and provided input during the evaluation to a standard of Proficiency.	Student conducted self in an appropriate manner, answered questions, and provided input during the evaluation to a standard of Adequacy.	Student failed to complete the interview or needs improvement in conducting self in an appropriate manner, answering questions, and providing input during an evaluation.	
Conclusion	Student has been recommended for continued employment and a 5% pay increase.	Student has been recommended for continued employment and a 3% pay increase.	Student has been recommended for continued employment and a 1% pay increase.	Student has been placed on 30-day probation.	
				TOTAL	

Based on the above criteria the student's grade for this assignment is: _____

(Total the points for each element scored and average for a final grade.)

Comments to the Student:

Instructor Signature: _____ Date: _____